HACK YOUR CHAKRAS

CREATE ENERGY FLOW, ENABLE VITALITY AND SELF HEALING

SUE FRASER

This book contains advice and information relating to health care. It is not intended to replace medical advice and should be used to supplement rather than replace regular care by your doctor.

It is recommended that you seek your doctor's advice before embarking on any medical program or treatment. All efforts have been made to assure the accuracy of the information contained in this book. The author disclaims any liability for any medical outcomes that may occur as result of applying any of the methods suggested in this book

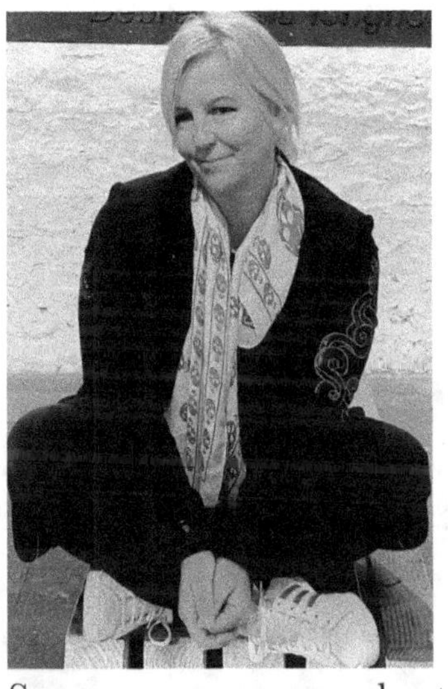

Sue Fraser has been a certified yoga, fitness, wellness and lifestyle coach since 2003.

During this time, she has coached over 40,000 people between her seminars, work-shops, coaching and training. She shares her wisdom and knowledge in what has helped her and her clients to create more energy, enable vitality and to self-heal.

Sue came across yoga due to a serious car accident in the early 2000 in which at the time gave her the time and space and to heal her mind, body and spirit in which it led to a path of self-discovery and her true calling.

In this guide Sue lays out simple tips to enhance your energy, vitality, and life force in which time will allow the healing to take place.

Namaste Sue Xx

CONTENTS

This book **"HACK YOUR CHAKRAS"** **Create energy flow, enable vitality and self-healing** contains proven steps and strategies on how to harness the subtle yet powerful life energy found in the chakras and use it to heal, balance and enhance your spiritual, mental and physical wellness.

This book contains the basic information you will need to understand what are chakras and how they affect you, as well as what the seven main chakra points are and what they are responsible for. You will also find simple and easy ways on how to balance and energize your chakras through simple meditation, colour meditation, healing foods, healing gem stones, essential oils and kundalini yoga poses, which is a yoga style that incorporates asanas (yoga movements) with mantra (chanting) and meditation.

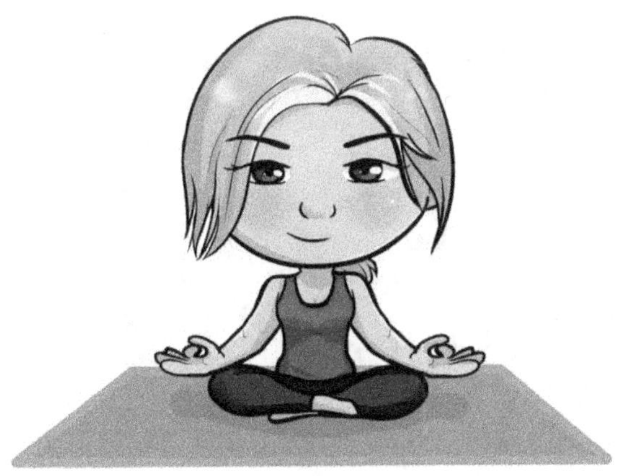

INTRODUCTION

To better understand what these chakras are all about, it is good to have a definition present. These are not just some types of energy centers though, they are ones that are found inside of your body and they are going to be in charge of regulating all of the processes that occur inside. This can include some things from organ function to your emotions and even how well the immune system works. For the most part, there are 7 main chakras and they are going to be positioned all throughout the body. Some people believe that there are some lesser chakras, but for now we are going to focus on some of the more familiar ones and how they are going to work in your body. These main chakras are going to be found from the base of the spine all the way up to the head and each one will have its own vibration, which is often shown with a specific colour that comes with the chakra.

Each of the chakras is going to work on a different part of the body. For example, the first chakra is going to be in charge of helping you to feel connections with the other people around you while the crown chakra opens you up to some of the things that happen in the spiritual world. All of the chakras are important, and they even work together, even though they may seem to work on such different parts of the body. When one of the chakras is not working properly, it can start to affect how the other chakras are going to behave as well over time. And if you don't take the time to give the chakras the healing that they need, you are going to start noticing that many of the chakras will start to fail. In addition, there are several ways that things can go wrong with the chakras. Many times, when there are issues, it is because the chakras are closed off and aren't able to let in some of the energy that is needed. For example, when the heart chakra is closed off, you may not be able to experience emotions and you may be seen as cold hearted to other people. In addition, you may find that the heart chakra, or any of the other chakras, could be too opened, which could result in you feeling too many emotions and always being a wreck from these emotions.

Chapter 1:

A BRIEF HISTORY OF CHAKRAS

As recently as thirty years ago the concept and knowledge of chakras were rare. Only a few people had heard of chakras and even fewer people practiced the lifestyle that comes with balancing and realigning your chakras. Now it is common knowledge and chakras are embedded into widespread media. The New Age of chakras comes with a lot of knowledge, ideas, and concepts that can be confusing and overwhelming to any newcomers and beginners. No matter how many different interpretations the new age chakra movement has brought, any beginner can join in on the lifestyle and reap the benefits that are on offer.

It may be a recent fad, but chakras are actually an old idea. It has changed slightly throughout the years as it has gone from one civilization to the next. For some it has become more complex. The main concept stays the same though. Before you can dive into the rich history of the creation of chakras and its development, you must first familiarize yourself with what a chakra is.

An Introduction to the Seven Chakras

The universe and everything in it are made up of energy. Our bodies are made up of and run on that same energy. This energy is a life force and ancient civilizations knew that this life force ran through everything in the entire universe. The energy connects us all. The seven chakras are not only part of this energy they also play an extremely important role in the natural flow of energy.

The natural flow of energy affects our mental, physical, and spiritual health. The seven chakras are the centers of the energy inside of us. The principle belief behind the chakras is that all seven of them must be fully balanced in order for us to stay healthy. The word chakra means 'wheel' or 'circle', as in a wheel or circle of energy. This meaning is based on the belief that the energy in- side you are constantly spiraling and spinning. Therefore, each chakra is at the center of the spinning energy. The positions of the chakras start at the base of the spine and carry on throughout your body all the way to the top of the head. The way the chakras are connected to your health is a simple concept. The energy inside you is al- ways spinning. In order for your mental, physical, and spiritual health to be balanced then your chakras need to be balanced. Your chakras are balanced when the energy in all seven chakras is spinning at the same speed and they are all perfectly in tune with each other. If one chakra is blocked and the energy isn't spinning, or if one chakra is being fed too much and the energy is spinning too fast, then all the other chakras are thrown off balance and your health are affected.

The easiest way to understand chakras is to imagine a river flowing through seven pools in your body. The seven pools of water make up the seven chakras. They are being fed by a waterfall which is the flow of energy from the universe. The energy runs through all seven of the pools from the top to the bottom. When the flow is calm and balanced all seven of the pools run smooth and their water is clear. However, water or energy is not the only thing that runs through the pools. Negative energy also runs through the pools,

this takes the form of dirt or algae. The negative energy flows into our chakras as easily as the positive energy from the universe does. It comes from things like stress, anger, and sadness which are things that are hard to avoid in life. When the negative energy gets too much, it starts to pile up inside our pools of energy and it turns the clear water into a dirty mess. Sometimes the dirt and algae block the flow of energy so that the water cannot properly flow from one pool to another. Even if only one of the pools is blocked the effects are seen in all seven of the pools.

In order for the water to flow through all seven chakras, we must clean away the dirt and algae. In other words, for our bodies to remain healthy we must clear away all the negative energy that is blocking our chakras. This is the only way the energy from the universe can flow evenly through all seven of our chakras. There are several techniques we can use to make sure our chakras are kept clean of any negative energy so our bodies remain healthy and balanced.

The Origin of Chakras

The origins of the Seven Chakras are India around 1500 and 500 BC. The oldest written tradition in India is called the Vedas and this is where the Chakra system was first mentioned. It was originally spelled 'cakra' but pronounced with a 'chi' like today's spelling for chakra. Although the words meaning was 'wheel' it was also supposed to be used as a metaphor for the sun.

The chakra system has changed hands throughout the years. It is believed that it was handed down through oral tradition by Indo-European people. These people were called the Aryan people. Until recently the chakra system was a tradition in Eastern philosophy. It has been brought to life and spread through current media as recently as ten years ago.

Since the New Age Chakra Movement and even earlier, the chakra system has been connected to many other forms of New Age health. Since the beginning, the chakra system has gone hand in hand with yoga and meditation. The chakra system is also connected to crystal healing, another New Age form of healthy living. Chakras are even believed to be directly connected to your diet and the foods you eat. The chakra system is a great lifestyle to follow. The benefits are well worth the work you put into it.

Chapter 2:

SIGNIFICANCE OF CHAKRAS IN OUR LIFE

We see the concepts of the chakras as an energetic system slowly permeate their way into the mainstream scope of the Western world from the Eastern world. The popularity of their significance appears amidst Yoga culture, in colleges and universities of the West for alternative medicine and healthcare practices, and the quickly spreading healing technique known as Reiki that originates from Japan also works with the chakras. They are the basis for working with the energetic system of all living things because not only do they appear in every living person, but also in animals. The chakras, originating from India in a developed medical theory over 2,000 years old called Ayurveda, were first written about in a thriving language during that time called Sanskrit. The term "chakra" is translated from Sanskrit to mean "wheel," as they are known to spin as energy passes through them.

In this first chapter, we will look at one of the most important aspects of the chakras, which is how significant they are. This is going to sound counterintuitive, since mostly what we hear is that any sort of unhappiness we feel is because of a problem in our life that causes us to be upset. But in reality, what happens is the exact opposite of that. The cause of our unhappiness from events happening around us actually originates from within us. That sounds confusing, right? How can we be upset be- fore we even have a problem? Well, this is how it works. Any problematic or potentially upsetting event that occurs in our life, like a disease of some sort or just general pain and discomfort, or even something like relation- ship problems and financial troubles, can be attributed to a problem that is already present somewhere in our body, whether it is from a physical, mental, or emotion- al aspect. Any such occurrence is merely a reflection of something knotted up or blocked that is already within us, but is something that we are not consciously aware of currently.

If you are having problems in your relationship with your partner, e.g. your girlfriend or boyfriend wants to break up with you, that breakup is actually because of a problem that was already present in your subconscious mind. A part of that feeling of separation comes from another part of you and has manifested as a problem: the breakup. It is like pulling away from yourself. But we humans tend to believe that the way someone else treats us should be a reflection of the way we treat ourselves.

This belief of ours will be reflected in our chakras, too. From the previous example of the broken relationship, the most noticeable effect will be on the solar plexus and the heart chakra. Besides that, the throat and the crown chakras will also be affected to varying degrees. Many organs and tissues in various parts of the body that are related to the chakras in question will be affected.

So how do we fix them? For this, we must first understand that healing is a process that occurs naturally and spontaneously if we only let it. Chakra meditation is how we heal our chakras and balance them. You do not have to fight the sensations you are feeling. You just have to let them flow. In the case of the previous example, you will feel some emotions and physical sensations because of the upsetting breakup. Here, the best course of action would be not to fight the emotions you are feeling, but allowing yourself to feel

them. With powerful meditation, you can let the sensations be with you and feel them, allowing them to be there with you fully. It becomes a practice of feeling and acknowledging your emotions without letting them over- ride or redirect your train of thought. If you are feeling poorly and you let those feelings begin to take your mind into poor and negative thoughts, then you are headed in the wrong direction. This will only make the situation clouded and more complicated.

Instead, you must attempt to focus on the sensation of the feeling by itself and feel it throughout your whole body, but without taking action or rather without reacting. You should allow yourself to cry if you feel the need to cry, and scream or shake your body in a safe place if you feel angry, without becoming violent. Any thoughts that come to you in this space should be allowed to pass through you like water through a running faucet.

When you catch yourself holding onto a thought in this state or getting carried away with it to other thoughts, you must work to let go of them as soon as you are aware that you are doing this and come back to the immediate sensation that you are feeling only. Any thoughts you have that spawn from the midst of an emotional state are driven by that emotion and thus are most likely to be distorted in some way because they are not coming from a clear mind. When you allow your thoughts to simply flow without becoming attached to them while you are feeling emotionally charged, you would eventually notice that your mind becomes clearer and calmer, and the emotion will finally subside.

Emotions are transient. They come and go like waves, and that is their true nature. The only reason that an emotion stays with us is because in some part of our consciousness, whether it be subconscious or otherwise, we are holding onto it. We hold on to the hurt, the anger, or the joy because it feels so real in the moment and it makes us feel validated as human beings, even if the emotion is an unpleasant one. We seek to justify those emotions with thoughts and reasoning, even if they are false because the emotion feels valid. When we come to understand the true nature of emotions as temporary sensations, we can learn to ride these waves in a healthy way for the moment that they surge or skim within us and then be done with them, ready for the next moment with a clear conscience. This is how you will be able to access the actual cause of your problem directly, which is the initial issue that caused the breakup. It could be some inner belief or some conflict within your mind, or anything else. Whatever it is, even if you are not aware of it, you can find this real cause of your problem and address it without thinking over and over again about suspicious reasons of your breakup. Your focus will be on the inner problem, not the outer one. I will teach you how to do that in this book.

Upsetting feelings and problems block our chakras from functioning and flowing smoothly, or they make them overactive if we end up holding onto those emotions and/or the thoughts that come with them from that initial experience, and the processing of it afterward. Both of these situations are bad. When you let yourself stay with the sensation and let the emotions flow through you freely, you witness a change. The chakras related to the problem begin to open up, and then start healing slowly. This happens automatically without you having to do much. That is the beauty of chakra meditation. And you will be astounded by this process each and every time, even if you have been

through it a hundred times. You will be amazed at your body's ability to heal itself if you just let it! It is awe inspiring really.

Sometimes an event in our lives can deal a blow so powerful and perhaps devastating that the sudden intensity of it prevents any possible processing from taking place. Usually, these are the ones where we have fully invested ourselves or simply left ourselves open and vulnerable, which is truly the way to get the most out of life, but the drawback that comes with these moments is we often walk away feeling damaged or broken from that blow. This can be a common sensation with relationship breakups or any stressful situation, especially if we do not see them coming.

People say that hindsight is 20/20, meaning that looking back at a situation is always clarified compared to being in the middle of it, although this is not the case when it comes to emotion. In the scenario just mentioned previously, the intensity of the event and the damaging sensation often stick with us for longer periods of time, and as we have discussed, the longer that emotions stick with us, the deeper they tend to get buried. It would be very difficult and require a skilled amount of processing with some kind of therapy to be able to clarify one's mind- set after such a blow in order to see a past event clearly enough to understand the situation and mindset as it truly was in that moment.

Many of us are accustomed to trying to think our way out of a problem using logic and reasoning. This can usually work when it comes to logical problems like accounting and business issues, however as a whole there is a lot more going on with us as human beings than logic and reasoning can find a solution to every time. In fact, some things, many things, run more deeply within us in psychological, emotional, and yes, spiritual ways than we often give them credit for. While we still may even have a sense of their presence to some degree, our overall awareness is limited to how far we are actually willing to go with it. In this respect, understanding the significance of chakras in our life comes with immeasurable value.

We all possess the capability of being financially successful in whatever way we are comfortable with that, along with developing harmonious and healthy relationships, including that most important one with ourselves which is intrinsic to the process, and we are all capable of learning how to manage our lives in a relatively stress-free way. Absolutely stress-free if you can believe it, and if you can- not, free in the sense that stress will not have the effect on you the way it does now. Instead, it will transform into a reminder of just what you are capable of and offer you a challenge to become even more. When it comes down to it, these things all depend on how much you allow your- self to have them and ultimately, it is how you look at it.

If you have not been aware, there is a kind of step- ping-stone effect related to our health and well-being that so far, I have alluded to in this book with conceptual examples. Medical science along with dozens of years of research in various types of psychology, psychotherapy, as well as metaphysics are all coming to understand and agree that physical ailments and symptoms of the body are indeed simply reflections of a deeper cause, which relates to stored emotions in our body. This phenomenon has been proven in studies on what is known as the somatic emotional response.

The next step in this method is the realization that, as we have been discussing, emotions that are stored in the body remain there and stagnate due to our mindset during and after the time that they occur. Our mindset is based on the way that we experience and perceive the world, and our individual perceptions determine what is stressful from one person to the next. This perception varies even within the same person from day to day. For example, if you start out your day feeling bad, you will be more likely to feel stressed throughout the rest of it, particularly by little things like a person cutting you off on the road. This heightened and lasting sense of stress, even if it is just triggered by small things, carries hormonal and chemical implications that are harmful to your body at heightened levels over moderate to long periods of time.

If you start out your day in a good mood on the other hand, you are much less likely to feel stressed, especially by some imperceptive person who cut you off on the road, but you will also be even more likely to accept challenging and difficult tasks throughout the day due to your personal sense of confidence and inner harmony. This goes to show, as more physicians and psychotherapists are seeing, that our health and sense of well-being is determined by our level of perception in how we see and experience the world. Those who perceive more things as being stressful will tend to be at greater risk for illness while those who maintain a healthy, rounded sense of perception will tend to be healthier overall. This goes further to show that just by working to change our perception to a positive one, or even a more neutral one, we are actively improving our health.

How do we help to improve our perception? There are many ways. We can become more informed by reading and educating ourselves. We can work to become less biased at large and see our world more objectively. And we can also monitor our thoughts to make notes on what tone they take on, where those beliefs come from, and if they are really our own or someone else's. Can you allow your beliefs to change to something more supportive? For yourself? For others? Would you make the effort to go ahead and make that change? Most importantly, though, tapping into our inner guidance and listening to it is the best source for improving our perception. The meditation practices that will come later in this book will help you to do that. From an improved perception, we improve our awareness of what is going on within ourselves as well as gaining clarified awareness of what is actually happening around us in the world. This heightened sense of awareness ushers in a higher consciousness that is brought forth in the alignment of all seven chakras.

This higher sense of consciousness will help to keep us aware of our thoughts so that they remain healthy, and when we keep a healthy mentality, we also keep our emotions in check. When our emotions stay balanced and we are able to ride their waves as they come with enthusiasm and compassion, our physical bodies benefit from this stability by maintaining good health. We can see though that from this progression, underlying causes of any illness always fall back from being strictly physical and they can almost always be healed from an energetic level.

As you will see in the following chapter, we have just successfully connected the relationships between the various bodies that make us up as human beings in the same way that the chakras align within us. From the first chakra being most related to the physical body and material things up to the seventh chakra correlating with our spiritual selves, more associations will be drawn to help you understand how to work directly and more in depth with the chakra system.

To review, the inner problems causing the outer problems in our life is usually referred to as an "upset," and in chakra meditation, we embrace the awareness of what- ever problem arises in our body and mind. This aware- ness alone leads to the gradual easing of the chakra or chakras affected by the upset. Once it is healed, it synchronizes with the other chakras and starts working like part of a great machinery, as it is supposed to. When all of your chakras work well together as a team, it brings inner peace and harmony. Your body starts radiating spiritual energy and balanced energy fields shift around you in a unified manner. These energy fields around us cause healing at the most organic and basic level. There is this innate intelligence within us that we are not aware of, and it can take care of everything once we start believing. Our mind and body start working as one once we embrace our inner conflicts and let our inner consciousness handle them on its own.

Chapter 3:

PRECAUTIONS WHEN OPENING CHAKRAS

While there is no need for you to fear any negative repercussions of chakra healing, it's useful to know a couple of guidelines to avoid pushing yourself too hard and applying the suggested techniques in the wrong way. The main risks from careless chakra healing arise from becoming obsessed with spirituality and lacking patience. Aiming to force yourself into spiritual growth can have harmful effects. A simple way for you to understand why, is to look at what would happen to your body if you would swallow a whole bottle of vitamins or take a double dose of a prescribed medicine. That would be a bad idea, right? Spiritual healing calls for the same amount of patience and honoring the body's natural pace as the common medical approach. This chapter will give you a couple of useful tips for smart and safe energy healing. This way, you will understand the importance of moderation, patience, and respect for the time it takes for your body and mind to heal.

Protecting Yourself When Working with Chakras

Chakra healing is universally safe and beneficial, if you stick to a couple of safety guidelines. Here's what you need to do for gradual and beneficial chakra healing (Govinda, 2004):

Don't Push Yourself

Balancing your chakras is all about patience and acceptance on all levels. Any intention to manipulate your body, mind, and energy may result in further energetic blockage. Expectations, on their own, are enough of a source of inner stress and tension. When practicing meditation, Qigong, Yoga, crystal healing, or using essential oils, make sure not to set any expectations of yourself. Chakra healing is all about letting go and accepting who you are in the present moment.

Release Judgment

Self-talk is an important part of reaching spiritual peace. It needs to be accepting and compassionate, not judgmental. Whether or not you reach any groundbreaking insights is irrelevant. What's relevant with chakra healing is to open yourself up for the inside messages. Just because you don't receive any signals or alleviation of symptoms right away, that doesn't mean it won't hap- pen during the next couple of days or even weeks.

Energy blocks are self-created, and it might take some time for the compassionate messages to sink in. The same way, it might take a while for your body to let go of negativity. Spiritual healing is largely an unconscious process, and while you may not feel any changes right away, they could be already in motion and waiting for the right time to manifest. Judging yourself for failing to see results is the same self-destructive pattern that caused the energy blocks to begin with.

Don't Set Goals

Unlike most worldly projects, the key to success with chakra healing is to abandon goal setting. Don't set goals or analyze and measure your progress. That being said, the measure of your success is the amount of openness, acceptance, and will to devote time to spiritual healing. Even this should be done with acceptance and compassion. Even if you encounter a block or unwillingness to do certain practices, you can use the experience to under- stand yourself better. For example, unpleasantness or resistance to meditating doesn't mean meditation isn't right for you. It means that you may be harboring fears of looking in or discovering something that you fear might be overwhelming. If this happens with any other technique, resort to mindfulness instead of worrying about slowing down your progress. Working around your fears and addressing them will be as beneficial as the healing technique itself.

How to Safely Use Chakras

Applying chakra balancing techniques is simple, and generally safe. Still, forcing your chakras to open up can be counterproductive. Your goal isn't to make all of your chakras hyper-productive, but to help them get back into balance and circulate your energy. To do this right, follow a couple of simple guidelines:

Get Professional Help

The same way your physical symptoms require medical treatment, so does your mental and spiritual symptoms. Make sure you are seeing reputable experts with a proven record of effectiveness. It's important not only for you to be safe, but to ensure that your practitioner has your best interest at heart. Aside from getting medical help for your illnesses, ask for all other help you can get.

For mental issues, see a reputable therapist. For spiritual guidance, consult a teacher within the range of your religion. For the purposes of using chakra healing, talk to those who share a level-headed, reasonable mindset. You will recognize a reliable spiritual practitioner by their simplicity, a realistic outlook on healing, and thorough knowledge of all aspects of the human body. A reliable practitioner won't discourage you from getting regular medical treatment, and they won't convince you to make irrational, unsafe life decisions. Instead, they will guide you towards measure and reasoning. For example, if you're looking to find balance due to a stressful job, a well-intentioned practitioner won't tell you to quit. Instead, they'll tell you that quitting would mean avoiding the problem and that the solution lies in developing emotional and spiritual tools to manage negative influences.

Kundalini Yoga and the Chakras

Kundalini energy, or evolutionary energy, is a powerful energy that all people hold in reserve in the base of the spine. This is considered as a powerful and also dangerous force that can cause illness, madness and discomfort if released when the body is still unprepared for it. Perhaps, this is why the visualization for kundalini energy is like coiled snake. However, there is a way to release or awaken kundalini energy safely, which can energize and open up your chakras. This is called Kundalini Yoga.

Kundalini Yoga is often referred to as the "Yoga of Awareness", and you can awaken it through meditation, pranayama or the extension of breath, chanting and Yoga asanas. Kundalini Yoga is about harnessing the power already within you and balancing out the chakras, a perfect way to get in touch with your center. All of this can be done in the comfort of your home all you need is a large bath towel or even better a Yoga mat. See the chapter on Seven Chakras it will give you some simple Kundalini Yoga poses that will help clear and open up the seven main chakra centers in the body.

If your aim is to heal or open your chakras, you need to visualize the colour that the healthy

chakra should have in order to complete the healing process. Also, if you find some of the poses difficult, don't push yourself or your body be- yond your limit.

Avoid Activating the Kundalini Energy Too Soon

The basic chakra system consists of seven chakras. These chakras each have a purpose in the body and are mutually connected. The three chakras in the upper body are spiritual and focus on connecting with your higher self and the Divine. Your higher self is a part of the purest manifestation of power, wisdom, and love. The three chakras in the lower part of your body are considered physical and tied to the Earth. Both spiritual and physical chakras connect in the heart chakra.

Aside from the seven chakras, there is also a source of energy called Kundalini energy. Kundalini is an enlightening force that has the ability to awaken all of your chakras at once. Every person has this energy. However, it's usually in a dormant stage, stored beneath the root chakra. Awakening of the Kundalini energy may happen suddenly, but that rarely happens. Usually, it happens after a long spiritual work, when a person has achieved enough balance, self-compassion, and acceptance. To awaken your Kundalini energy, it is best that you work slowly and practice at your own pace. Once you manage to awaken it, you'll feel a sense of electricity climbing from the root of your spine to the top of your head. This process can be cultivated with Kundalini yoga or regular energy work.

You should aim to activate your Kundalini energy safely, gradually, and with proper guidance. If you do the process right, the awakening of Kundalini energy will bring you joy, bliss, and healing. It will awaken your psychic and intuitive sensibilities. There are some health repercussions to awakening your kundalini energy suddenly. If you awaken your kundalini under the influence of others while you're not fully prepared, your energy can get stuck between your root chakra and your crown chakra. From this, many painful symptoms can arise that will be hard to manage. This can lead to both emotional and mental instability. If you've awakened your kundalini energy spontaneously, ask for the help of both physical and mental health experts to get back into balance. To add, there are more ways to awaken your Prana and balance chakras without awakening your kundalini energy. There are other ways that are more subtle and safer, long-term, compassionate, and patient work to get both your body and mind into balance.

Chapter 4

BENEFITS OF A BALANCED CHAKRA SYSTEM

Throughout our lives we are put into situations that cause us physical trauma or distress, emotional instability, and leave us mentally drained and spiritually stunted. This can put a stop to your life. Feeling this way could also make your push your friends and family away. All of this can lead to a downward spiral where you feel lost, as if you don't know who you are anymore and you don't know why this is happening to you. One of the reasons that you feel like this could be because one or more of your chakras is unbalanced.

When one or more of our chakras is blocked, then energy cannot freely flow through us. Often when a chakra within us is blocked, a part of our life is left blocked as well. This can lead to many unhealthy and bad effects to our minds, bodies, and souls. This is why it's important to unblock and balance your chakra system. Remember that your chakras are like pools of water in your body and they are all connected and flow through each other, so even if only one of your chakras is blocked it will throw all of the chakras out of balance and start affecting you.

Besides feeling happier, healthier and more in tune with yourself and the universe there are many benefits to balancing your chakra system. Each chakra is blocked by a specific thing and each chakra brings something to your life if they are balanced. Here I will describe the overall benefits you will achieve when you have all seven chakras balanced.

Amazing Benefits of Balanced Chakras:

1. Unblocking your chakras will also release blocked emotional and physical energy. Blocked emotional energy could lead to unresolved feelings of sadness or vulnerability. Unblocking this energy will make you feel happier, more energetic, and less vulnerable.

2. Blocked chakras can lead to confusion and difficulty with understanding simple tasks and solving problems. Unblocking your chakras will leave you feeling more motivated and confident. You'll be more likely to succeed in all your endeavors and reach your goals.

3. With unblocked chakras you will feel and look younger, and you will feel healthier than ever before.

4. You will feel more in touch with your intuition. Blocked chakras can make you doubt yourself and feel negative about your thoughts and feelings. With balanced chakras you will trust your intuition more and no longer doubt yourself.

5. You will feel a stronger emotional connection in your relationships. Having balanced chakras allows you to be more in touch with your emotions which will let you feel things more deeply. Although you will be more connected with your emotions, you will be in full control so you won't be overwhelmed by them. Having a balanced chakra system is just one step towards fully con- trolling your emotional state and being able to connect to others' emotions in relationships.

6. Lying is something we all do. Whether it's to save ourselves from embarrassment or save someone else from being hurt. However, if your chakras are balanced, you will be able to understand the importance of the truth better and you will be able to express the truth easier. You will also be more understanding when hearing the truth from others, even if it is a hard, cold truth.

7. You will be more comfortable and self-confident. It's no secret that we all feel a little insecure in our own skin. Having a balanced chakra system can fill you with confidence and help you be more comfortable with yourself and even with your own sexuality.

8. Balancing your chakras can even lead you to have a better memory.

9. A balanced chakra system can give you more energy and motivation. This can help you with weight loss among other things.

10. Balancing your chakras can help you connect to your subconscious mind. This has many benefits on its own, along with feeling more aware.

11. Balancing your chakras can help you rid your life of many things that plague us all: stress, anxiety, insomnia, depression, addiction, and so on. Having a balanced chakra system means having a balanced life.

12. Having a balanced chakra system will allow you to think more clearly and will even promote creativity.

13. You will have more mental toughness. This means that you will be able to withstand more abuse and hurt from the world. The world can be harsh and any number of things can leave us feeling hurt and broken. Having a balanced chakra system will allow you to be able to withstand the world's harsh ways and will leave you feeling more capable to fight against or ignore it.

14. With balanced chakras your overall health will improve and your immune system will be more capable of fighting back against illness. When

your body is in harmony you are healthy and strong. When your body is disorganized and unbalanced you are left weak and open to illness. If you balance your chakras and your body then you will be healthy and stay healthy.

These are simple benefits that come from a balanced chakra system but they can lead to you feeling like a new person. You will feel like you can do and handle anything life throws at you. There are many things we do in modern times that we weren't meant to do. We weren't meant to sit in an office all day long and work. We aren't supposed to be stressing about a hundred different things all at once. We weren't meant to spend our lives working in order to survive. This is why so many people live with unbalanced chakras. This is why so many people today are sick and tired all the time. There are so many parts of the modern world that can lead to our chakras being blocked and unbalanced. The modern world is designed to unbalance us. We can fight back by putting ourselves first and focusing on balancing our chakras. Once your chakras are balanced you will be more equipped to handle the things in life that are set to unbalance us.

Negative Energy Versus Positive Energy

What exactly unbalances our chakras? The answer is simple; negative energy. The universe is filled with energy, both negative and positive. Energy from the universe flows into us. The positive energy flows through us freely but the negative energy cannot flow as easily. It is more likely to become stuck inside of us if we do not know how to release it properly. When the negative energy starts to pile up, that is when the natural flow of positive energy is stopped and our chakras are blocked. The differences between positive energy and negative energy are many. However, the main difference between the two is how each of them enters our bodies. Once again, the universe is filled with energy but our bodies willingly let the positive energy in. We do not willingly let the negative energy into our bodies. The negative energy forces its way into our bodies through certain events.

Negative energy thrives in traumatic experiences, emotional hurt and mental challenges. Things like pain, whether it's physical or emotional, invite negative energy into our bodies. Stress, anxiety, self-doubt, hatred, anger, depression, addiction, loathing, and jealousy are all part of the flow of negative energy. These are the things that invite negative energy into our bodies and the negative energy becomes stuck inside our energy pools if we don't have the tools or knowledge to release it properly. We are not all born with the ability to properly release negative energy from our bodies. Things like traumatic life experiences are difficult to live through and even more difficult to let go of. Something as simple as being yelled at by your parents for breaking a dish can send negative energy into your body. When we were children, we didn't know how to properly understand and release this negative energy. Chances are that that negative energy is still inside of you. This is how easily our chakras can become blocked by negative energy. The more it builds up, the worse it can be for your health and the harder it will be to release it.

Although this knowledge may seem overwhelming and it may make you feel hopeless, there is still a reason to have hope. We are all born with the ability to take in positive energy from the universe and give positive energy back to the universe. Understanding, identifying, and releasing negative energy is something we need to learn. Identifying the negative energy is always the first step. Now that you know what negative energy is and where it comes from, you are already on your way to learning how to release it properly and unblock your chakras. Once you learn to release the negative energy inside you and your chakras are balanced, you will see that it is not as easy for the negative energy to enter your body as it was before.

Chapter 5

THE SEVEN CHAKRAS

You would often hear the word "chakra" when you are speaking with a spiritual healer, chiropractor, acupuncturist, or a yoga teacher. But it's a word that's not commonly used in this modern world. In fact, the word "chakra" does not appeal to a lot of people because it sounds too "hippie" or "new age". Many people think that these chakras are not real and that they do not exist. But chakras are real and they have a huge impact in your life, whether you believe in them or not. They influence the level of your energy. They also govern your emotions, your health, and even the quality of your life and relationships. But what are chakras? Where are they located and why should you care about them? Chakras are energy centers or fields of the body. These energy fields, primarily operate on your spirit or non-physical body, but they do correlate with areas of the physical body.

The chakras are wheels that move the energy up and down the body as they spin. They are connected to specific

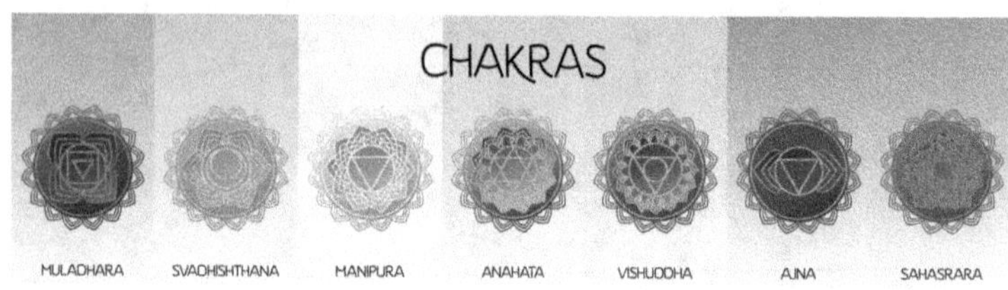

organs and glands in the body and they are responsible for the distribution of the life energy called "chi/qi" or "prana". The chakras are the foundation of your energy ecosystem. Problems or deficiencies in this ecosystem can negatively affect the different areas of your life. When one or two of your chakras are blocked, you'd experience health and mental issues. There are many energy centers in your body, but there are seven major chakras that are located from the base of your spine to the top of your head.

Root Chakra (Muladhara)

The root chakra is the first chakra it gives us a sense we are grounded and connected to the environment it also taps into our instincts for survival, self-preservation instinct and fight and flight.

This chakra is very active in your first 7 years of your life. It is the densest of all the chakras. The chakra is associated with our sense of smell a great way to enhance it is through candles, incense, essential oils around your home, massages, going out in nature, sitting on grass or under a tree to absorb the earthy energies, cooking, body oils and creams.

Element: Earth

Location: Base of spine, right above our tailbone

Colour: Red

Physical Level: Bladder, hips, legs, vertebral column, adrenal glands, kidneys, low blood pressure, anemia, digestive or bowel problems.

Signs of Balanced: Feel secure, stable, full of health, energy, vitality, full of strength.

Healing and Balancing Gemstones: Red jasper, black tourmaline, blood stone, red carnelian, obsidian.

Essential Oils: Embodies the frequencies and healing properties of plants it helps to balance and heal the physical, emotional, mental and spiritual.

Sandalwood, myrrh, frankincense, cedar-wood, ginger, lavender, cinnamon, ylang ylang.

Healing Nutrition: Red Foods, pomegranate, red-currants, strawberries, raspberries, cherries, red apples, watermelon, tomatoes, peppers, radish, beetroot, chili peppers, cranberries, pink grapefruit, red kidney beans, red grapes, red plums, rhubarb, guava, radicchio, red onions.

Blockages:

This chakra is extremely sensitive. This chakra represents security and stability. When this chakra is blocked, you'd experience the following symptoms:

☐ Kidney infections and Anemia

☐ Tumors in the rectal area
☐ Reproductive health issues
☐ Laziness
☐ Addictive behavior
☐ Circulatory issues
☐ Bladder irritations
☐ Anxiety and depression
☐ Anger and rage
☐ Low self esteem
☐ Leg and lower back pain
☐ Fear of change and stubborn
☐ Materialism
☐ Lack of energy and motivation
☐ Insecurities

When you feel a lot of these symptoms, take time to sit down, breathe, and say these affirmations.

☐ I am grounded.
☐ I am safe.
☐ I am powerful.
☐ I am brave.
☐ I have enough.
☐ I am centered.
☐ I trust myself.
☐ I am open to possibilities.
☐ I am loved.
☐ I am willing to change
☐ I trust people.
☐ I nurture my body with clean water, food, exercise, and water.

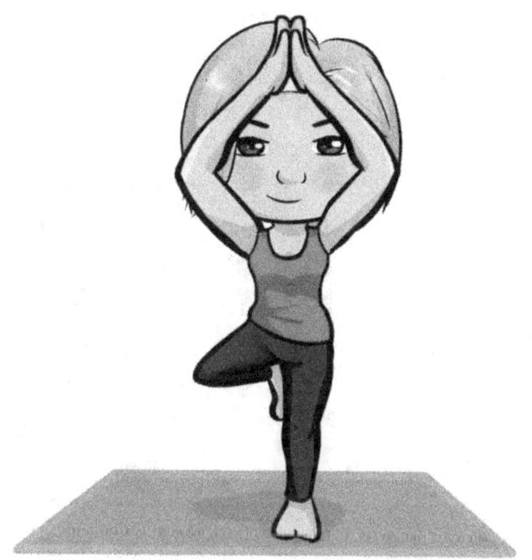

Tree Pose (Vriksasana)

Vriksasana, which literally translates into tree pose, is one of the well-loved yoga poses or asanas across different generations of yogis. In fact, the creation of the pose can be traced back to prehistoric India. It is called as such because, just like a tree, you are supposed to stand and sway gently when the wind blows or when other distractions come your way. Ideally, you should also do this pose with a tree next to you. By doing so, you can link to the energy of the trees by touching or hugging them.

It primarily benefits your root chakra where your memories when you were young are kept. One of these memories is about whether or not your basic necessities were given back when you were a child. You can unblock and balance it with the help of the tree pose.

Steps:

- ☐ Decide whether you want to do it outdoors or indoors. If you want to stick to traditional yoga and make the most out of the tree pose, you should practice it near a tree. Doing the pose indoors will also do just fine. It might help you concentrate better if you are doing it indoors.
- ☐ Stand up with your arms resting on your sides. Your weight should be equally distributed to your feet. In yoga terms, this standard position is known as the Mountain Pose or Tadasana.
- ☐ Transfer the weight from your right foot to the left. Then raise and bend your right knee. Your right sole should rest on your left thigh or ankle, but never let it rest on the left knee. Make sure your left foot is directly below the center of your hips. Adjust your left foot and hips accordingly.
- ☐ Let your hands stay on your side for a while. Next, put your hands together akin to a praying position with your thumbs in front of your sternum and your hands in front of your heart chakra. Focus your vision into one stationary point in front of you.
- ☐ Press your left thigh (or left ankle) and right sole evenly against each other.
- ☐ Breathe in as you raise your hands with your palms still pressed together.
- ☐ Stay in this position for a minute. Step back and return to Mountain Pose to release the pose. Repeat the steps on the opposite side for the same amount of time. Repeat 3–5 times each side.

Sacral Chakra (Svadhisthana)

The sacral chakra is the second chakra it connects to our feelings, emotions, sexuality, creativity and our relationships with other people and the world. Sometimes known as the partnership chakra. The emotions, fears, and strengths associated with this chakra drive your behavior. When this chakra is balanced, your body moves freely and easily. You also enjoy good health, strong in- tuition, compassionate and emotionally stable. You are motivated and focused in pursuing your personal goals.

Element: Water

Location: Below the navel and above the pelvic bone.

Colour: Orange

Physical Level: Uterus, sexual organs male and female, intestines, lower sacrum, bladder.

Healing and Balancing Gemstones: Red garnet, jasper, carnelian, citrine, shungite, tangerine quartz, gold- stone.

Signs of Balance: Enthusiastic, happy, energetic, sporty, self-assured, constructive, living in a state of grace, flexibility and sexual fulfillment.

Essential Oils: Orange, ylang ylang, neroli (flower of the orange tree), sandalwood, jasmine.

Healing Nutrition: Orange foods, almond, papaya, melon, passionfruit, oranges, pumpkin, mandarins, mangoes, walnuts, coconut, sweet potato, squash, carrots, seeds for their good fat, wild caught salmon.

Blockages: But when this chakra is off, you'll also feel that something's not right in your life. It could lead to various symptoms such as:

- ☐ Guilt, jealousy and lack of motivation
- ☐ Infertility issues and menstrual issues
- ☐ Low back pain, diarrhea and diabetes
- ☐ Low libido and inability to orgasm
- ☐ Depression and low self-esteem
- ☐ Detachment and aloofness
- ☐ Lack of vitality
- ☐ Lack of flexibility
- ☐ Weight loss and loss of appetite
- ☐ Chameleon personality and bipolar mood swings
- ☐ Lack of focus and poor boundaries
- ☐ Immobilized by fear and fear of change

When your sacral chakra spins too fast, you often experience jealousy, mood swings, and sexual addictions. You often consider people as sex objects and you may be overly dramatic. If your sacral chakra is underactive, you may have digestive disorders and sexual issues. You may be oversensitive and shy. If you're overly shy or you've been acting like a drama queen lately, then you should say the following affirmations daily.

- ☐ I am confident.
- ☐ I am comfortable with my sexuality.

☐ I accept myself.
☐ I am at peace.
☐ I am radiant.
☐ I listen to my own truth.
☐ I respect my emotions.
☐ I have the capability to provide for my own needs.
☐ I trust my instinct.
☐ I am enough.
☐ I am graceful.
☐ I am creative.
☐ I am grateful for everything in my life.
☐ The universe is filled with beauty.

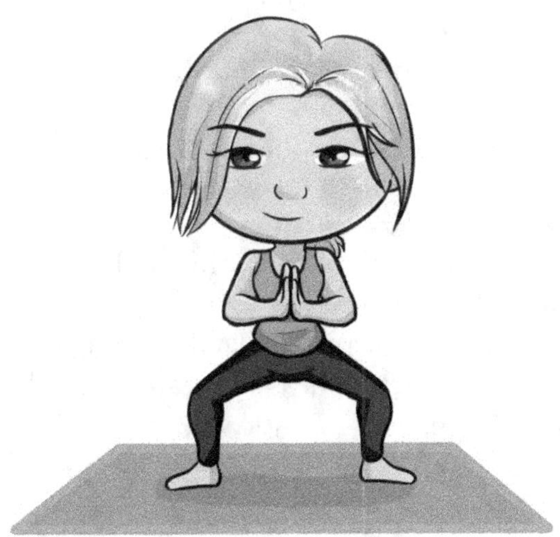

Goddess Pose (Utkata Konasana)

Utkata Konasana which literally translates into goddess pose, is known by other names such as: victory pose, Fiery Angel. Even though it is named after a female, males are allowed to practice and make this pose a part of their routine.

The goddess pose opens your sacral chakra which is responsible for your emotional stability and creativity. The pose also strengthens your sexual energy which can positively affect your fertility. Additionally, it makes your thighs and calves stronger and more toned.

Steps:

- Begin with the Mountain Pose (feet firmly planted on the ground, feet parallel by keeping toes together and heels slightly apart, belly drawn into your spine, neck neutral, shoulders back and relaxed. Next, stretch your feet about four feet apart. Ex- tend your toes outward and then inhale deeply.
- As you exhale, bend your knees and make sure your thighs are parallel to the ground.
- Stretch your arms to the sides with your palms facing downwards. They should be at shoulder level.
- Slowly press your palms together near your chest.
- Soften your shoulders as you stare at the skyline.
- Hold this position for at least 30 seconds. Increase the duration to a minute once you are flexible and strong enough to do so.
- Slowly lower your arms whenever you feel discomfort with this position.
- Return to the Mountain Pose to release the Goddess Pose.
- Repeat the steps 4 to 5 times.

Solar Plexus Chakra (Manipura)

This is the third chakra known as the jewel of the navel connects to our ego, will, personal power and autonomy.

This chakra is your energy center and it radiates energy throughout your whole body. It is where we gain a mental understanding of our emotional health and is responsible for our will power. Balancing this chakra makes you feel centered in spirit, body, and mind. It also helps you get more connected with your intuition or gut feelings so that you may act accordingly and with confidence. Heat is your solar plexus friend, so hot yoga, walk in the sun- shine, sit in front of an open fire or spend time in an infrared sauna helps balance it out

Element: Fire

Location: Upper abdomen or the stomach area, between the rib and the navel.

Colour: Yellow

Physical Level: Spleen, liver, small intestine, pancreas, diabetes, low blood sugar, muscular stiffness, poor digestion.

Signs of Balance: High self-confidence, childlike energy, they are open minded, stress free, respect authority, strong sense of community and team spirit, they are also practical and intellectual.

Healing and Balancing Gemstones: Malachite, topaz, citrine, amber, tigers' eye.

Essential Oils: Peppermint, clary sage, lemongrass, Fennel, coriander, lime, frankincense.

Healing Nutrition: Yellow foods, corn, squash, beans, bananas, brown rice, millet, pineapple, quinoa, amaranth, spices, ginger, turmeric, yellow peppers, complex carbohydrates, oats, potatoes, white bread products, white rice, lentils, chickpeas, lemons, chamomile.

Blockages:

If this chakra is unbalanced, you're overly critical and judgmental. You'll easily find fault in others. You may be demanding and may have extreme emotional problems. You may be rigid and stubborn. You are also more likely to engage in a codependent relationship. You'll also experience the following symptoms:

- ☐ Diabetes and constipation
- ☐ Binge eating and obesity
- ☐ Lack of self-control
- ☐ Gallstones
- ☐ Hepatitis
- ☐ Inability to lead others
- ☐ Stomach ulcers and pancreatitis
- ☐ Allergies
- ☐ Reflux problems
- ☐ Inability to reach goals and self-esteem issues
- ☐ Growing addiction

When your solar plexus chakra is not balanced, you can say the following affirmations.

☐ I am strong and powerful.
☐ I am empowered.
☐ I make my own choices.
☐ I treat myself respectfully.
☐ I trust myself.
☐ I am worthy of love and kindness.
☐ I am authentic.
☐ I direct my own life.
☐ I am at peace with myself.
☐ I am responsible for my life.
☐ I release my desires and appetite to the universe.
☐ I accept my responsibilities.
☐ I make my own choices.
☐ I am successful.
☐ I am in control.

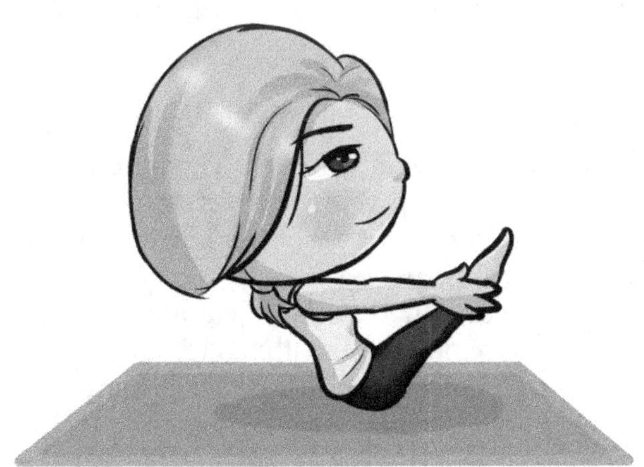

Boat Pose (Navasana) — Strengthening the Navel Chakra

The boat pose, or Navasana in yoga terms, is named as such because you are supposed form the letter V akin to that of a boat. It has two types namely the full boat pose (Paripurna Navasana) and the half boat pose (Ard- ha Navasana). The full boat pose requires you to fully extend your legs and arms while the half boat pose allows you to bend your knees.

Of the two types, the full boat pose is the one recommended for the solar plexus chakra.

It strengthens the lower back and abdomen.

The boat poses are not suitable for those who are suffering from hypotension, diarrhea, or headaches. You have to work your way out of such conditions first before you can practice either the full or half boat pose. ***The poses are also not recommended if you have asthma or a heart problem. Furthermore, if you are currently menstruating, you are not supposed to do either boat pose.***

Steps:

- ☐ Sit on the floor with your knees bent and your feet on the floor. Keep your back straight. Your hands should be resting at your sides with your palms facing downwards.
- ☐ Inhale and exhale slowly, calmly and evenly. Concentrate on your breathing.
- ☐ Lean back little by little. Slowly lift your feet. Your shins should be parallel to the floor.

☐ After that, lift your feet and draw your lumbar region in. Stretch your arms forward with your palms facing each other.

☐ Keep your back straight. Do not let your chest collapse. The area below your navel should be somewhat flat and firm but not thick and too hard.

☐ Beginner level just go to position 3 and if you need to hold onto your legs. Immediate and advanced straighten your legs as you exhale. Your body should now form the letter V as you stretch your legs.

☐ Keep your breathing calm. Stare at your toes. Concentrate on your awareness.

☐ Hold the position for five breaths or up to a minute. To release, breathe out while you bring your feet and arms to the floor.

Heart Chakra (Anahata)

The heart chakra is the fourth chakra connects to our emotional self, bringing harmony, forgiveness, sincerity and love. It also governs our ability to give and receive unconditional love. This chakra connects the lower to the higher chakras and is vital for self-healing and self-development. The heart chakra is where we find true self love and when we can truly love ourselves we then can love others. A tip to keep well is to eat or drink green plants in which brings micro pranic energy vibrations and when this chakra develops into full bloom its light frequencies gradually change and reflect the pink light of unconditional love. This chakra is also associated with the thymus gland an organ which is vital in children's immune system.

Element: Air, walking in nature helps to balance it.
Location: Centre of your chest.
Colour: Green.

Physical level: Immune system, lungs, thymus, heart, blood circulation, premature ageing, upper back problems, pneumonia, asthma, respiratory problems, heart palpitations, poor circulation, difficulty in breathing.

Signs of Balance: Compassionate, caring, adapt to change easy, calm, friendly, fun, cheerful.

Healing and Balancing Gem Stones: Green jasper, emerald, jade, green tourmaline.

Essential Oils: Ylang Ylang, rose, jasmine, pine, rosewood.

Healing Nutrition: Green foods, spinach, kale, limes, cucumber, lettuce, cabbage, broccoli, leeks, celery, green apples, pears, kiwi, green grapes, avocadoes, matcha, mint, Asian greens, beans, peas, spirulina, wheatgrass, green tea, all green herbs.

Blockages:

Holding a grudge or a traumatic event may block your heart chakra. Repressed feelings can also negatively affect the function of your heart chakra and can lead to:

☐ Loneliness and feel unworthy of love
☐ Social anxiety and shyness
☐ Holding grudges and fear of getting hurt
☐ Inability to give or receive freely

☐ Fear and suspicion in romantic relationships and friendships
☐ You are extremely self-centered and easily lose your patience
☐ You feel embarrassed of your failures
☐ You have difficulty breathing and you have allergies
☐ You have heart and lung issues

When you have an overactive heart chakra, you are unable to say no to others. You try your best to please others and you are desperate for other people's love and appreciation. When you have an underactive chakra, you feel like you're cold, shy, and resentful. The heart chakra controls most of your emotions. So, if you want to achieve emotional stability, it is important to keep this chakra balanced. These will help heal your emotional wounds. If you have problems giving and receiving love, say these affirmations aloud looking in the mirror, in the morning after you wake up and at night before you fall asleep.

☐ I love myself just as I am.
☐ I forgive myself and I forgive others.
☐ I trust in the power of love.
☐ My heart is filled with love.
☐ I open my heart to unconditional love and respect.
☐ I love my life.
☐ I am compassionate.
☐ I openly receive love.
☐ I am not afraid to love.
☐ I am grateful.
☐ I embrace and open my heart to love.

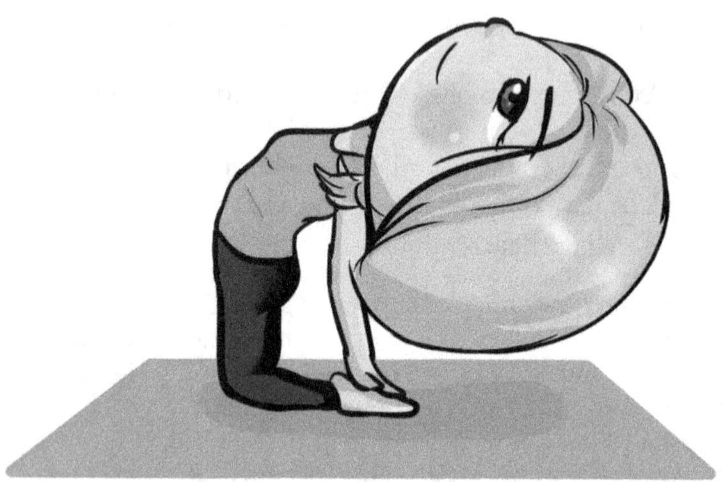

Camel Pose (Ustrasana)

The camel pose has many health benefits that are widely recognized. In fact, this particular pose has been ad- opted by nearly every type of yoga routine. This pose opens and heals the heart chakra, and balances the navel chakra. It is also good for overall health as it strengthens immunity and builds strength. ***Please be careful ifyou have a weak back.***

Steps:

- ☐ Sit up on your knees that must be hip width apart. Your toes should be flat behind you.
- ☐ Tilt back, your face turned upwards, extend your chest place your hands on your lower back for support and arch your back. ***You might only be able to go this far and that is perfectly fine***

until you build up the strength and practice if you can carry on as your hand reaches down to hold the heels of your foot. Your hips should be pressed forward. If this is too difficult tuck your toes in. Slowly release using your hands for support stretch up to the sky and then do a lower back stretch.

☐ Do the breath in this pose for about 30 seconds to a minute, and gradually extend the time until you manage to hold the pose for 7 minutes.

Throat Chakra (Vishuddha)

This chakra, as the name suggests, is located at the throat. This chakra keeps us well by constantly bringing subtle energy vibrations from the earth's atmosphere and sky into our physical body. Its main aim is to purify. When this chakra is balanced you will have the ability to speak your truth. Nature is a great way to help balance, blue skies, singing a song out loud, calling a friend, or writing a letter.

Element: Natural Element of Ether or Akasha meaning the infinite space, sky or atmosphere.

Location: Throat

Colour: Aqua, turquoise

Physical Level: Associated with respiratory system, gums, mouth, teeth, thyroid and parathyroid glands, exhaustion, body weight being too high or low, thyroid, throat and neck issues

Signs of balance: Self-expression, creativity, truth, communicate your beliefs, ideas, emotions.

Healing and Balancing Gem Stones: Aquamarine, turquoise, blue quartz, blue tourmaline.

Essential Oils: Black spruce, cedar, eucalyptus, lavender, fennel, ginger, jasmine, myrrh, rosemary, spearmint can use with oil burner, diffuser or bath.

Healing Nutrition: Blue foods, blueberries, a lot of water, fruit teas, soups, blackberries, blackcurrants, apples, pears, eggplants, figs, plums, prunes, purple potatoes, rai- sins, purple cabbage, lemons, limes.

Blockages:

Habitual lying is not just a character flaw, it is also a symptom of blocked throat chakra. Throat chakra blockage has also a number of other emotional and physical symptoms such as:

- Extreme shyness
- Social anxiety
- Inability to express thoughts
- Inconsistency in actions and speech
- Stubbornness
- Inhibited creativity
- Detachment
- Chronic sore throat and laryngitis

☐ Frequent headaches
☐ Mouth ulcers
☐ Thyroid problems
☐ Neck pain
☐ Hoarseness

People with blocked throat chakra are deceptive, manipulative, domineering, anxious, and insecure. So, if you're constantly insecure or envious, take time to say the following affirmations.

☐ I have a voice.
☐ My opinions matter.
☐ I speak the truth.
☐ I uphold the truth.
☐ I am free of all delusions.
☐ I claim my voice.
☐ I am speaking my personal truth.
☐ I let go of the chains that are holding me back.
☐ I have a beautiful voice.
☐ I am not afraid to speak my feelings.
☐ I listen to others.
☐ I am content and truthful.
☐ I value honesty.

This yoga position is excellent for promoting brain health and brain function. It also calms the mind and brings forth peacefulness. This pose also massages the neck and opens up the chakras. ***Please do not do this full version if you have any neck, lower back or shoulder problems.***

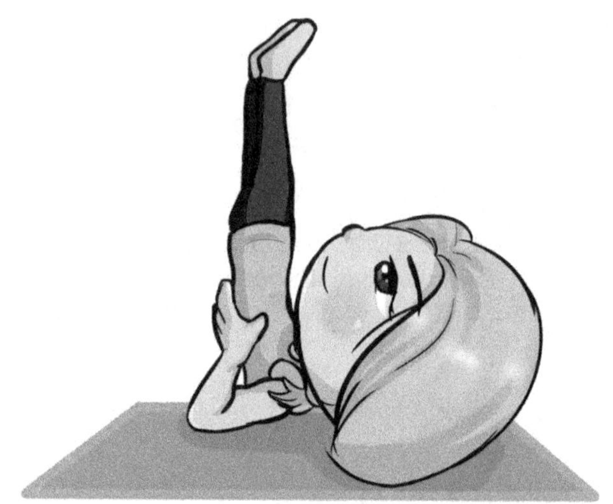

Supported or Shoulder Stand (Sarvangasana)

Steps:

- ☐ Start by lying flat on your back.
- ☐ Raise your knees to your chest then extend them. With your elbows flat and pointing slightly outward, forming a sort of triangle, put your hands to your waist for support.
- ☐ Lift your waist off the floor until your weight is supported by your shoulders. Try to extend into as much of a straight vertical position as possible.
- ☐ Start to take long, deep breaths. Hold this position for 15 seconds minimum. Gradually extend the time you hold this pose until you can hold it for five minutes.
- ☐ If you have a sore neck or shoulders lie flat on your back and just stay in position 1 or lie against a wall and evaluate your legs against the wall.

Third Eye Chakra-Brow (Ajna)

This chakra is the sixth chakra it represents our ability to see the big picture and make sound decisions it's about your intuition and imagination. This chakra balances your circadian rhythms of sleeping and waking. This chakra also unlocks psychic powers of telepathy, clairaudience, clairvoyance and access to past lives.

Element: Light

Location: Forehead between the eyes

Colour: Indigo-Blue

Physical Level: Eyes, face, parts of the brain, lymphatic system, endocrine system, bouts of dizziness, extreme nervous and anxiety, being over analytical, need external stimulants to keep you going, feeling cut off from your life purpose.

Signs of Balance: Trusting your abilities, following your dreams, being in touch with your intuition, having the ability to be decisive, consciousness expands, we become unattached to material possessions, fame or fortune and have no fear of death.

Healing and Balancing Gem Stones: Purple amethyst, tanzanite, indigo, sapphire, satyaloka quartz, celestite.

Essential Oils: Holy basil, frankincense, jasmine, geranium, lavender, rosemary.

Healing Nutrition: Purple foods, figs, blackberries, purple carrots, purple potatoes, eggplant, grapes, raisins, prunes, purple kale, purple asparagus, cardamom, ginger, mint, nutmeg, sage, turmeric.

Blockages:

Third eye chakra blockage can wreak havoc to your health. It could disrupt your day and it could lead to serious mental issues. It's normal to feel crazy on some days. But, if you're feeling crazy too often, then you may have a blocked third eye chakra. So, if you feel that your intuition is out of whack or you get deceived easily, you may be experiencing third eye chakra blockage. If your third eye chakra is blocked, you'll experience these symptoms:

- ☐ Poor vision and migraines
- ☐ Seizure
- ☐ Sciatica
- ☐ Inability to focus
- ☐ Oversensitivity
- ☐ Delusions and paranoia
- ☐ Depression and anxiety
- ☐ Fear of success and pride
- ☐ Lack of clarity and discipline
- ☐ Cognitive problems and psychotic behavior

If your third eye chakra spins too fast, you're proud, dominant, manipulative, and you may be living in a fantasy world. If it spins too slow, you're often confused. If you experience any of these, by saying these affirmations you will begin to heal this chakra.

- ☐ I see clearly.
- ☐ I have a strong intuition.
- ☐ I have an open sixth sense.
- ☐ I am important.
- ☐ I am intelligent.
- ☐ I am open.
- ☐ I am ready to see the truth.
- ☐ I am wise.
- ☐ I trust my intuition.
- ☐ I forgive myself for my past.
- ☐ I accept myself.
- ☐ I am open to bliss and inspiration.
- ☐ I am at peace and I release my past.

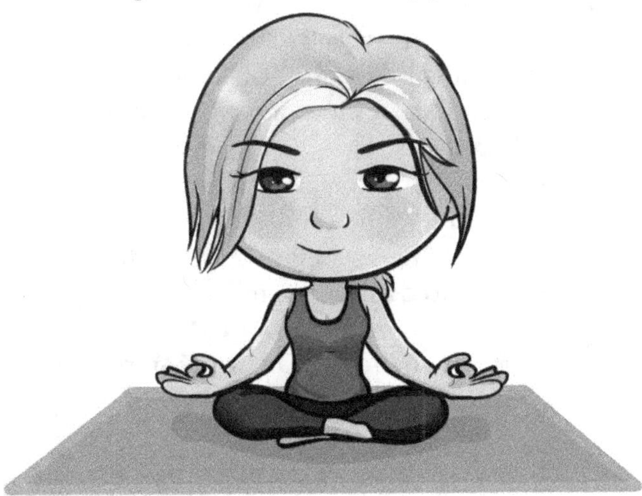

Third Eye Meditation

This meditation technique opens up the brow chakra, develops intuition, and willpower. It is even believed to help you develop psychic powers. Also, this meditation can improve vision and breathing.

Steps:

- ☐ Sit on your heels with your arms raised up in a 60-degree angle, palms facing upward. ***If this position is difficult for you, you can sit in a simple cross-legged position or on a chair.***
- ☐ The breathing is in counts of 16, which is related to the third eye, 16 inhalations and 16 exhalations in tiny breaths.
- ☐ Visualize a small silver hammer lightly tapping the center of the forehead. Keep your gaze fixed on the center of your forehead. Look up to the center of your brow then close your eyes.
- ☐ Now breathe in 16's. ***This is the difficult part*** and it will take all of your focus and concentration. Remember to be patient with yourself in this. This is a difficult meditation practice and you must be patient with yourself as you do this.
- ☐ Do it for a minute and gradually lengthen the time that you take to do it. Remember not to strain your eyes when you turn them toward the center of forehead. It is better to just start with your eyes closed in the beginning.

Crown Chakra (Sahasrara)

This chakra is the seventh chakra. It represents your spirituality and it allows you to experience pure bliss or pure consciousness. Sometimes people have a negative experience with religious institutions, or experience trauma in their life, and this blocks any connection to that higher being. If you are too bossy or find yourself at high end department stores, you have an unbalanced crown chakra. So, when you start to balance all your chakras and being to make peace with your past only then can you really begin to heal.

Element: Ether or Space (Spirit).

Location: Top of your head.

Colour: Violet, gold, white

Physical level: Brain, nervous system, pineal, pituitary glands, disturbing psychological disorders relating to past karma.

Signs of Balance: Understand things in a wider context, you feel you are in the right place at the right time, feel empowered, at peace, enlightenment, great energy and joyful.

Healing and Balancing Gem Stones: Rainbow quartz, amethyst, black merlinoite, clear quartz, sugilite.

Essential Oils: Lotus, linden.

Healing Nutrition: As this chakra is more spiritual than physical it's not nourished with food but **in** the same way it is connected to all the other chakras, so please keep in mind when choosing food keep it Pure, Non-GMO, Organic.

Blockages:

- It can also lead to a number of symptoms including:
- Loneliness and lack of direction
- Inability to build a genuine connection with others
- Inability to set and maintain goals
- Nerve pain
- Learning difficulties
- Indecisiveness
- Lack of inspiration and joy
- Confusion and delusions
- Over intellectualism and dominance
- Nightmares and amnesia
- Epilepsy and brain tumors

Having an underactive crown chakra leads spiritual addiction. This means that if you're a "know-it-all", your chakra may be spinning too slowly. This is the reason why you should make sure that your crown chakra is balanced. You can also say the following affirmations to help balance your crown chakra.

- I am complete.
- I am one with the Divine Energy.

☐ I am a spiritual being.
☐ I believe.
☐ I go beyond my limiting beliefs.
☐ I am aligned with the Divine Energy.
☐ I am wise.
☐ I am open to questions.
☐ I understand.
☐ I am open to enlightenment.
☐ I am open for pure bliss.
☐ My consciousness is growing and expanding.
☐ God's love heals me.
☐ I am open minded.
☐ I accept myself totally.
☐ I feel pure joy.

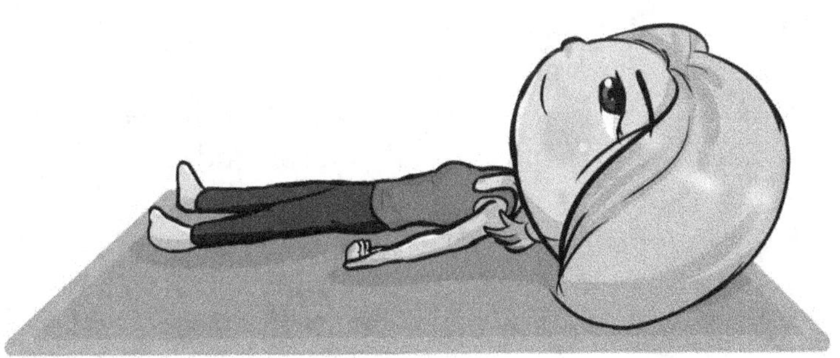

Seventh Chakra — Unlocking the Crown Chakra

The name comes from the Sanskrit words shava meaning "corpse" and the Asana meaning posture, Shavasana is the simplest and the main relaxation pose used in yoga. It is performed at the beginning and at the end of yoga practices. It is also used as a resting pose between other asanas. The benefits include reduction in the rate of breathing and metabolic rate and fatigue, decrease in general anxiety and panic attacks. Increase in memory, focus and concentration levels. Relaxes the mind and body giving a sense of wellbeing.

Steps:

- ☐ Sit on the floor or your mat with both feet flat on the floor with your knees bent, using the arms gently lie on the floor lowering your back flat down, place your body in a straight line, palms facing up and relaxed. Arms rest away from your body. Slide heals one at a time extend your legs, spread comfortably apart and close your eyes and allow your body "melt" into the mat or floor feeling all points of contact.
- ☐ If this position is difficult for your back keep your knees bent or roll up a large towel and place under your knees.
- ☐ The emphasis is given to slow, rhythmic and relaxed breathing, the breath is done with full awareness.
- ☐ As your breath in one expands the abdomen first, then the chest and then the neck region sometimes known as three phase breathing. When breath out,

the process is reversed, the neck and chest region contracts first and finally the abdomen.

☐ After a few breaths when you start to feel relaxed and the mind stays aware. The breath will eventually become shallow, at that point, just the abdominal

☐ breathing takes over. You can maintain this position for 3–30 minutes.

☐ *To release this position, take a few deep breaths, stretch your arms over your head stretch your toes down, imagine two people are stretching you clasping your hands and ankles, slowly draw your knees into your tummy clasp your knees and slowly roll your lower back for side to side give yourself a big "HUG" and thanking yourself for spending the time on doing this practice. Roll to the side and very slowly guide yourself up using your arms to a seated position.*

New Emerging Chakras

The root chakra, solar plexus chakra, sacral chakra, heart chakra, throat chakra, third eye chakra, and the crown chakra are the seven major chakras. But some chakra systems actually have 12 chakras, which include the earth star chakra, navel chakra, causal chakra, soul star chakra, and stellar gateway.

Soul Star

The eighth chakra is called the soul star chakra. This chakra cleanses and heals your lower body. It is located around eighteen inches above the crown chakra. This chakra is known as the seat of the soul. This chakra governs your life purpose.

Earth Chakra

The earth chakra is the ninth chakra. It is located one foot below the ground. This chakra keeps you connected to the earth. It is the center of a powerful force called Kundalini.

Solar Chakra

This is the tenth chakra. This chakra attaches you to the angels that dwell in the sun. This chakra plays an important role in spiritual evolution.

Galactic Chakra

This chakra is hooked up from the palm of your hand and it is linked into the galactic system. So, if you want to get the best out of life, you should try to clear your energy centers and make sure that they are functioning correctly.

How Chakras Work

We all have a physical body and we also have an energy body. Our energy body contains our auras and meridian lines. Auras are non-physical energy fields that surround a person. Your aura reveals your thoughts, dreams, and feelings. The colors of your aura may vary and they are usually seen by people who have special training in the healing arts. A meridian line, on the other hand, is a path where the life energy called "qi" or "chi" passes through. It is a typically used in Chinese medicine. If you go to an acupuncturist or a spiritual healer, you'll hear these terms often.

When you cut the body open, you won't see these auras and meridian lines, but you know that they are there. When you are familiar with auras, you'd know that they are affected by certain vibrations good or bad. So, if you get a good vibe or bad vibe from someone, you may be feeling his aura. You get certain feelings when you talk with someone because these vibrations are contained in their energy. Like the auras and meridian lines, the chakras are part of the body's energy anatomy. They operate like a ball of energy and they spin like a wheel to distribute your energy evenly throughout your body.

You can't see these chakras through an X-ray because they are not part of the physical body. They are part of our consciousness and they interact with the physical body through the different organs in the body. Each chakra is associated with one endocrine gland and a group of nerves called plexus. As mentioned in the earlier chapter, there are seven major chakras or energy centers. Are some chakras more important than others? The answer is no. All chakras are equally important. To live a good life, you should balance all the chakras in your body.

The grounding function of the root chakra is just as important as the spiritual function of the crown chakra and the transcendent quality of the heart chakra. To optimize your mental and bodily functions, you have to balance all your chakras and address your basic, relational, creative, safety, belongingness, and self-actualization needs.

The Chakras and Your Physical Body

We are all made of pure energy. So, if your energy centers are blocked, you'll experience various illnesses. When one or two of your chakras are not spinning, the energy is not evenly distributed throughout your body, resulting to some of organs may not functioning well. For example, your heart chakra is in your chest area and it covers the heart, and the respiratory system. So, if your heart chakra is not spinning, you'll experience heart and circulation problems. You are also susceptible to respiratory diseases and allergies.

The throat chakra governs the throat and mouth area of your body. So, if it's not functioning well, you'll experience mouth ulcers, sore throats, and thyroid problems. Many Western medical practitioners do not believe this, but your chakras can affect your body functions. Balanced chakras can optimize your health and vitality while unbalanced chakras can wreak havoc in your life.

Chakras and Emotions

Chakras do not only represent your physical body, but also your emotions and parts of your consciousness. When there is tension in your consciousness, you'll feel it in the chakra that's linked to that part of your consciousness. For example, if your boyfriend leaves you, you'll feel the pain in your heart or chest area. You'll feel like you can't breathe. When you are nervous about something, your bladder becomes weak and your legs tremble. When the tension persists, it can result to physical symptoms.

The Chakras and The Quality of Life

The chakras do not only affect your physical body, they also affect your mental health and the overall quality of your life. So, if one part of your life seems off or something in your life is not working, then one of your chakras may be blocked. When one or two of your chakras are blocked, some parts of your life may be doing well while other parts of your life may not be doing well at all. For example, your career may be doing well, but you have difficulty maintaining healthy relationships. If you are a spiritual, kind, and compassionate person, but you have a hard time paying your bills, you may also have blocked chakras.

When your chakras are not functioning the way they should, you feel there is an imbalance. Your subconscious tells you that something is amiss. The chakras represent who you are your intellect, emotions, creativity, spirituality, sexuality, careers, principles, and your belief system. So, if your chakras are not balanced, you'll lose sight of one part of your life. You'll likely develop psychological problems such as depression, anxiety, delusions, and even nervous breakdown.

What Causes Chakra Blockages

Chakra blockages are caused by several factors *belief system, career, living situation, financial situation and relationships.* Traumatic experiences such as abuse, accident, and loss of a loved one may also cause chakra blockages. Negative emotions such as anxiety, anger, stress, and fear may also put your chakras out of balance. For example, being physically and emotionally abused by a former partner may cause heart chakra imbalance. You might have ended up closing your- self out to potential romantic partners. You may also tend to feel empty most of the time. Your root chakra represents the foundation of your being. So, if your parents do not have enough money when you were growing up and they failed to provide enough for you, you'll most likely experience root chakra blockage. You may constantly fear that you do not have enough. You may also constantly worry about money.

Opening and Closing the Chakras

The opening and closing of your chakras work a lot like an energetic defense system. When you experience something traumatic or negative, the associated chakra will close itself to keep the negative energy out. If you are clinging to low frequency feelings such as anger, guilt, or blame, you'll experience chakra blockage. Holding on to the following low frequency emotions for a long period can cause chakra blockage:

☐ Anger
☐ Pain

☐ Resentment
☐ Jealousy
☐ Covert hostility
☐ Grief
☐ Apathy
☐ Hopelessness
☐ Sadness
☐ Regret
☐ Pessimism
☐ Worry
☐ Blame
☐ Discouragement
☐ Shame
☐ Powerlessness
☐ Depression
☐ Disappointment
☐ Frustration
☐ Despair
☐ Guilt

The following positive or high frequency emotions can raise your vibrations and help open your chakras:

☐ Love
☐ Joy
☐ Acceptance
☐ Eagerness
☐ Optimism
☐ Passion
☐ Hopefulness
☐ Contentment

☐ Faith

☐ Belief

So, to keep your chakras balanced, you must let go of egoism. You must choose to act with love. You should also consider trying various chakra healing tools which will be discussed later in this book.

Chakras and Empaths

Many people have open chakras. These people are called empaths. They are highly sensitive people. They easily pick up other people's energy so they find public places overwhelming. They also know when someone is not being honest with them. They are creative and they have a strong need for solitude. They feel weak when they are exposed to toxic people. Empaths should keep their chakras guarded and balanced. They should carry protective stones such as rose quartz, black tourmaline, amethyst, and malachite. These stones help balance emotions and remove anxieties and negative energy.

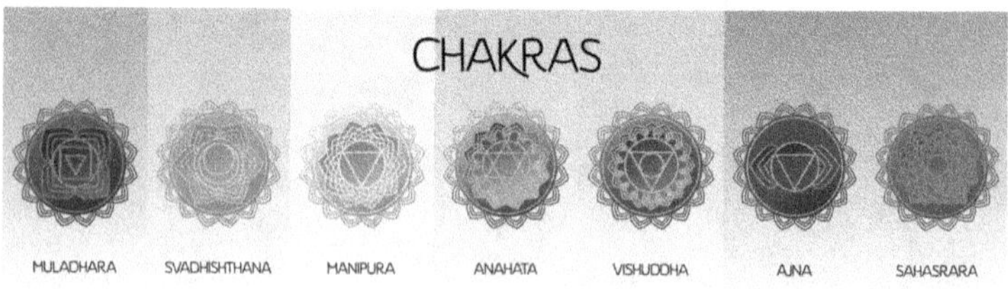

Chapter 6:

CHAKRAS AND WELLNESS

Now that you know the right ways to balance your chakra, the next step is to learn how to maintain permanent spiritual wellness. Spiritual wellness entails continuous spiritual health. Without commitment to permanent changes, you could easily fall out of balance again. This chapter will further reflect on meditation and the ways in which you can use it to heal your chakras. Moreover, the sections of this chapter will provide you with ways to use meditation to look inside so that you can nurture and accept your inner being. The following chapter will further explain the meaning of spiritual wellness and suggest the techniques that you can incorporate into your daily life to maintain peace, accept and listen to your chakras, and stay balanced (Sherwood, 1988).

Using Meditation for Chakra Health

Meditation is best done by sitting in the Indian or the lotus position. Since the root chakra is located at your tailbone, this position will allow you to feel the roots of your body. This way, the meditation will lead to an increase in your sense of grounded-ness and stability.

Grounding Meditation

Your root chakra is associated with your faith into being provided with the essentials in life beyond what manifests in the physical world. This means that a true sense of safety isn't conditioned by the proof you see on the outside. Meditating on the root chakra increases your sense of stability, and as a result, leads to more financial stability and confidence in your ability to make money. This allows you to feel safe regardless of circumstances and helps you overcome problems. With a stable root chakra, you'll feel like the Earth is always supporting you. You'll never feel insecure.

Sacral Meditation

Your sacral chakra is located below your navel, and it is a source off of selflessness, pleasure, and graciousness. Sacral meditation will make you more charitable and open to give to the world. It will enforce your connection with the world, with those close to you, and the less fortunate. A balanced sacral chakra decreases depression and the sense of loneliness. Meditating on your sacral chakra will increase your awareness and sharpen your intuition. It will also sharpen your ability to have knowledgeable insights.

Solar Meditation

Your solar plexus chakra is located in the upper abdomen. It's in charge of self-confidence and control. When you are disengaged from your solar plexus, you will feel a lack of confidence and an extreme desire to be in control. A disengaged solar plexus can give you a feeling of butterflies in your stomach. This is the sign that your chakra is feeling weak. Often, placing your hands upon your stomach signals nervousness. It is a sign that the area is being overstimulated. By regularly meditating on your solar plexus chakra, you will increase your confidence in both yourself and the world. As a result, you will feel better connected, and your overall sense of trust will increase.

Heart Meditation

Your heart chakra is in the center of your chest. Meditating on it helps you gain the ability to love, both yourself and others. It will allow you to find inner peace, as well as to experience and express joy. The heart chakra meditation has many physical benefits, such as the regulation of your heart rate, blood pressure, and cholesterol.

Throat Meditation

Your throat chakra is located directly in your throat, but it also connects with your sense of hearing. This chakra is in charge of your sense of balance and the ability of communication. A balanced throat chakra enables you to express yourself and be open to listening to others. It can be very helpful for you to release negative thoughts that have been building up by verbalizing them and speaking them out. Meditating on the throat chakra and maintain its health ensures that you feel more comfortable expressing your fears and voicing insecurities. It increases your creativity and will to be a good listener.

Third Eye Meditation

Your third eye chakra, also known as the brow chakra, helps you focus and see the big picture of your life and the world around you. Taking good care of this chakra will help you manage daily stress and inner pressure. Meditating on the third eye chakra enables you to surpass and overcome past trauma and difficult memories. It keeps you in touch with the source of your intuition and wisdom. Being in tune with your third eye chakra will constantly remind you that the world is an abundant source of love and all kinds of riches.

Crown Chakra Mediation

The Crown chakra sits at the top of your head, keeping your body connected to the spiritual. It completes the system of seven chakras that starts at the base of your spine. Your crown chakra is the gateway for your Prana, or life energy of your body. It is the place where life energy enters your body. Meditating on the crown chakra opens your mind to both exterior and interior peace. The crown chakra stimulation will bring you calmness and relaxation. When you meditate on the crown chakra, you will feel a strong connection with God or whichever source of power you believe.

Practices to Utilize the Chakras for Wellness

Getting in touch with your chakras means getting in touch with your inner, invisible, energetic self, that communicates unconsciously. Connecting with your chakras enables a fully fulfilled life, heals illnesses, and creates a holistic approach to healing inside-out. Using mindful- ness and meditation, you can strengthen the connections between your body, mind, and spirit.

How to Get in Touch with Chakras

To connect with your inner energy, you should hold your hands an inch apart from one another. Familiarize yourself and feel the warmth of energy that is being exchanged between the palms of your hands. To do this, relax and clear your mind. When you start feeling the energy between your hands, you can proceed to stretch it by separating your hands or flex it by joining your hands. After repeating this for a couple of times, you will be able to notice a gentle energy charge between your hands. The longer you exercise, the more you'll feel the intensity and the warmth of energy increasing. You can apply the same process to feel your chakras.

To start feeling a chakra, place your hand onto the desired area of your body. It can be either the top of your head, the area between your eyes, your heart, the areas above and beneath your navel, and your pubic bone. Take a deep breath and feel the warmth underneath your hands starting to intensify. You will feel the area pulse, and you'll feel your blood flow both in that area and in your hand. If that doesn't happen, be patient and repeat the process a couple more times. Chakras are the energy centers that help you develop self-consciousness. Your aura is often referred to as the eighth among your chakras, and your third eye chakra visualizes your spiritual insights. It accesses your spiritual truths. The third eye's power lies in the intuition, and it's often associated with the pineal gland.

Evaluate the Health of Your Chakras

You can check your chakras to see whether or not you have a healthy flow of energy through your spine. A trained practitioner will be able to tell you which of your chakras are underactive and which are overactive. Both overactivity and under-activity are harmful because they put you in a state of imbalance. Aligning your chakras can be done in many ways. Some of the techniques you can practice to align your chakras include eating foods that fuel them, doing exercises, taking relaxing baths, and doing other things that either open up or calm down your chakras.

When talking to practitioners about balancing chakras pay attention and make sure their intentions are pure. Pay attention to only a reputable expert. Many internal and external factors can contribute to the misalignment of the chakras. The chakras process the experiences and the information that enters your being. Then, they use physical signals as a way of communicating these experiences to you. Some of your behaviors and physical symptoms can relate to over or under-activity of the individual chakras.

Accept and Surrender to the Messages

Learning how to accept and surrender to receiving all the signals that your chakras are trying to send will help you balance them. Ignoring your feelings causes energy blockage, which leads to many diseases and ailments that result from energy disruptions. When you're unaware of the importance of energetic alignment, you are often treating the symptoms, externally through traditional medicine. This is a superficial approach that is as effective as, for example, fighting a fire by extinguishing the fire alarm. Aside from getting the right medication for the diseases, you should also pay attention   to the health of your energy body. The purpose of everything you do to align your chakras, from meditation to reiki, Qigong, and other practices, is to open your chakras to either start receiving energy or to release the excess energy.

Overactivity of the chakra means that it keeps receiving energy, but it's unwilling to let it go. An underactive chakra is closed to receiving energy. Either way, the best way to balance your system is to open the chakra, to either release or start receiving energy.   Spiritual wellness helps you develop an interpersonal connection between yourself and the Universe in a way that is harmonious. It entails exploring your own sense of purpose and meaning. There are many ways to do it. You can use mindfulness, affirmation, prayer, yoga, and other exercises that connect you to your inner and higher power. These practices mainly target your belief system, because beliefs are the root cause of all of your troubles. All blockages and self-imposed limitations come from predominating negative beliefs. When you start working towards establishing positive beliefs, you will move towards trust and safety. You will find it easier to work around fears and insecurities.

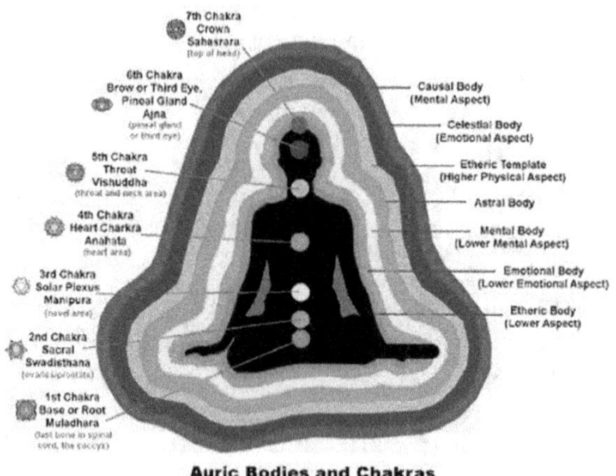

Auric Bodies and Chakras

Chakra with Colors

Colours have a lot to do with chakra healing, the brightness and dullness of a colour has a certain effect on us mood, with certain colours associated with warmth and energy while other colours associated with coolness and calm, and everyone has their own preference in colour. But how can colours have such a strong effect on chakra healing? Every colour has its own wavelength and frequency and has a different effect on people. This chapter will be devoted to the colours and the different ways you can make use of colour to heal, uplift and energize your chakras.

The Colours

Red – Root Chakra

Red is the colour for the root chakra and is widely viewed as the symbolic colour for bravery, love and life. This colour stimulates energy, brings warmth and helps you get connected to the root chakra.

Orange – Sacral Chakra

Orange, the next colour up the spectrum, is a lighter version of red. It stimulates balance and sustains warmth. It can enhance sexuality, creativity and make you more sociable. It can even bring about happiness and make you more receptive to pleasures.

Yellow – Solar Plexus Chakra

The color associated with the sun, yellow, brings light energy into the body. It energizes and brightens the aura and it can help when you are engaged in grueling physical activity. Working on this energy chakra and colour enhances well-being and creativity.

Green – Heart Chakra

The colour green is associated with the heart chakra and is a colour that can soothe the mind, body and spirit. To the mind, green can be the most relaxing colour. Green enhances the connection between man and the earth and of new life. A combination of cool and calming blue with the energy and life of yellow, green is the most balanced of all the colours. Visualizing breath in the colour green maximizes healing and meditation. Visualizing this colour associated with the heart chakra enhances focus, builds up compassion and empowerment, balances the energy and uplifts the mood.

Blue – Throat Chakra

Blue is a colour that calms and relaxes both body and mind. It generates expansive energy that helps with relaxation. Blue is associated with thoughtful and deep love that is spiritual in origin. A good colour for healing, especially in children, it is a good colour for the home if you want to enhance calmness and quietness in the mind. Envisioning this colour can help in the peaceful and truthful expression whether it is with words or in song.

Indigo – Brow Chakra

Often considered the colour of royalty, indigo is associated with spiritual and higher consciousness. It has a deeply calming, almost tranquilizing effect, but it can cause depression if there is too much. This colour, when associated with the brow chakra, can develop self-esteem, discernment, wisdom, develop intuition and give you clarity.

Purple/Violet Chakra — Crown Chakra

Considered to be the colour of transformation, violet is a calming colour that can help control nervousness and promote relaxation. You can also use this colour to build up self-esteem. Working on the crown chakra with the colour purple can stimulate dreams, bring clarity and connect you to your higher consciousness and spirituality.

Harness the Power of Colors

There are many ways to harness the power of colours and let them affect and change your energy levels, clear your chakras, balance your energy and change your mood. Before embarking on this journey of colour healing, try to review the different emotions associated with the different chakras that have been mentioned above. You will need this knowledge for you to know what chakras to work on during your therapy.

Chakra Balancing Colour Therapy

Step 1: As per the usual, find a place where you can relax and not be disturbed for fifteen to thirty minutes. It has to be somewhere you are comfortable in and won't feel insecure or on your guard.

Step 2: Have seven pieces of cloth that correspond to each of your main energy chakras ready. Lie on your bed or the floor. Make sure that you can hold this position for 15 – 20 minutes without getting hot or cold.

Step 3: Relax. Close your eyes and take several slow deep breaths. With every breath, feel your body relax further.

Step 4: As you begin to feel your body relaxing, reflect back on your day in reverse, starting with when you laid down for your chakra colour therapy, to when you woke up this morning.

Step 5: As you reflect on every moment of your day, think of the emotions you felt and the part of the body that felt affected. Identify what emotion it was you were dealing with and if you felt any physical pain that you associate with this type of emotion.

Step 6: Try to identify which chakra vortex was affected by this or that particular emotion. If needed, you can use a table or a list of emotions that particular chakras are responsible for.

Step 7: Once you have completely evaluated yourself and your chakras, it is time to start the colour therapy. Open your eyes slowly and take the cloth that corresponds to the chakra center that you believe need energizing and place this over the corresponding main chakra center.

Step 8: Now, with the coloured pieces of cloth over your main chakra points, it is time to visualize. Close your eyes and breathe deeply. As you take long slow breaths, feel the colour from the pieces of cloth being absorbed by your chakra and drawn into the body. Start from the highest point. For example, if you feel deficiencies in your throat, navel, and root chakra, start with your throat, then go down until you reach the lowest point.

Step 9: As you visualize this, feel your energy centers balance out and become re-energized. Feel the corresponding organs and organ systems become active and vital, feel your chakras balance out.

Step 10: Continue this visualization technique for 5 - 10 minutes or until you feel balance as a whole and feel your ailments dissipate. Repeat these steps as needed (whenever you feel an imbalance in your body or if you feel a little emotional etc.).

Chapter 7

HEALING THROUGH YOUR CHAKRA

Using the methods of chakra healing, you can treat numerous physical ailments that weren't caused by medical problems or injuries. Pain and diseases that root in mental causes, instead of medical, are called psychosomatic. They are called this because they signal mental distress. They are a sign that your body is overrun by stress hormones and fear hormones. However, it's not enough for you to acknowledge that some of your ailments come from your mind. To understand which particular aspects of your emotional life are struck with blockage and denial and to learn how to release them, you can look into each individual symptom and tie it to the corresponding mental problems. The following sections will explain the most frequent psychosomatic symptoms and how they relate to chakras (Permutt, 2015). With this information, you'll understand your body better, and you'll know which of your symptoms result from emotional and spiritual problems.

Headache

If you're suffering from chronic headaches without obvious medical causes, it could be due to the imbalance in your third eye chakra and the crown chakra. Chronic headaches, followed by sinus pressure, and the pressure in the back part of your head and your eyes, that spread across your forehead, are the most typical sign of the dis- harmony in the third eye chakra. These pains are a signal that you are mainly focusing on the intellectual and neglecting the spiritual aspects of your existence. You may be afraid of your spiritual aspects. Because of this, you are ignoring your intuitive hints and abandoning the wisdom of your third eye. Many times, your instincts tell you to do things that seem to go against logic. You feel these signals, but you are afraid that acting on them would be risky. For example, if you unconsciously feel like you should quit your job, but there is no new job in sight, you might be ignoring this instinct.

Subconsciously, your third eye knows the things that are beyond your conscious knowledge. It might be signaling to you that the better opportunity is coming your way. Or, you may be in the presence of a person you unconsciously know has a negative effect on you. But you are ignoring the intuitive signals to stay away from that per- son. On the other hand, a headache at the top center of your head is often a sign of the imbalance in the crown chakra. This type of headache suggests difficulty trusting the intuitive signs regarding your life path. You may fear that acting and living in accordance with the Divine signals will lead to something risky or irresponsible. This results from having difficulties in seeing a larger picture and cultivating your faith in yourself and in the Divine.

Fatigue

Fatigue is detrimental to your energy focus and concentration which all results in low motivation. If you are someone who usually overwork themselves into exhaustion, you are overloading your solar plexus chakra and your power center is being overstimulated. If you're suffering from fatigue, it is most likely due to the imbalance in the crown chakra and the solar plexus chakra. The ongoing exhaustion that only increases and doesn't go away after rest, with a constant feeling of weariness and low energy, signals chakra imbalance. This can happen if you are associating achievement and self-esteem with the quality of your performance. If you feel like failing to deliver quality performance makes you unworthy, it can have a negative effect on your solar plexus chakra. This is often followed by low self-esteem, depression, and loss of faith in the Divine.

Stomach disorders

Pain and uncomfortable symptoms in your stomach come from the imbalance of the solar plexus chakra. Diseases related to stomach include diarrhea, constipation, intestinal problems, ulcers, acid reflux, and many others. If you are certain that you haven't eaten any foods that might have upset your stomach, or that there haven't been any physical injuries that might have caused these symptoms, you can inspect your solar plexus chakra to see if it's out of balance. Pain in your stomach can often result from the feeling of powerlessness, a sense of overwhelm, a perception that you are losing control of your life, feeling intimidated or having low self-respect. If you went through significant changes in your life, like a divorce, problematic relationships with other people, or a loss of a job, these experiences could have produced a lot of anger, resentment, guilt, and other toxic emotions. If your self-esteem is compromised, you will have a very toxic combination of negative feelings towards other people and yourself. The key to resolving this is to forgive both yourself and others, as well as admitting that there is no reason to place blame on anyone.

To overcome stomach pains related to the solar plexus chakra, you can apply the solar plexus meditation or use essential oils to treat your stomach area with more kindness and compassion. Psychosomatic digestive problems arise from your problems with processing stress. They are a sign that you are ignoring to resolve problems in your daily life. When you're not processing daily stresses, they become suppressed. You are resorting to emotional avoidance. As a result of this, you are closing your solar plexus chakra because you don't want to deal with problems. This is dangerous because your solar plexus is the center of your personal power. When you avoid confronting problems, you are shutting yourself out from using your personal power to solve them. As a result of this, you feel frightened, powerless, and your self-esteem is low. The only solution for this is addressing the things that are bothering you.

Detachment

When you feel disconnected and detached from yourself and the world around you that means that you've closed your heart chakra. In this state, you abandon your passions and you give up everything that makes you happy and fulfilled. The first sign of the imbalance of the heart chakra is the lack of connection with others. You may feel the need to be alone, which can turn into isolation. When you feel the need to isolate from others, it means that you are shutting yourself out. You want to feel happy and joyful, but it seems like you are no longer able to.

You are out of touch with everything that makes you happy. This can lead to depression. You may even be disconnected from your physical body and unable to feel the physical sensations before they become overwhelming. For example, you don't notice symptoms of illnesses before they become too intense. You start living on autopilot, disengaging from your true self. Detachment is best treated with mindfulness. Start looking into every- thing that makes you happy. Focus on gratefulness and put more effort into spending time with your friends and family. First, you need to establish a good connection with yourself, which can be done through meditation and other self-care practices.

Depression

While physical trauma can induce depression, it is mainly a mental state in which a person's negative beliefs prevail over the positive perceptions of oneself and life. What gives people a sense of purpose, meaning, and a feeling that they belong in the world is faith in God. Having faith in God is essential because none of us are truly in control over anything, including our own lives and our own bodies. What keeps us going is the faith that there is general positivity in the world and that things will work out for us. We rely on this faith even when outside manifestation speaks otherwise. Due to traumatic events, a problematic childhood, or a combination of multiple factors, negative beliefs can prevail over positive thoughts. When you have experiences like these, your heart chakra and your crown chakra will fall out of balance. Your heart chakra is in charge of being open to love. It is in charge of feeling worthy of love and wanting to love others selflessly and unconditionally. Related to that is the crown chakra, which embodies your relationship with the Divine.

That relationship is primarily a relationship of love. It requires faith. When you fall into depression, you essentially lose faith in love. Not only in love, you lose faith in "good," which resonates with losing faith in God. This is an unconscious process that might not manifest in conscious thoughts due to blockage. You don't want to admit that you've lost your faith and you block out these feelings. As a result, you feel hopeless and undeserving of anything good. In this state, both your crown and heart chakra will close or constrict. You will experience continuous sadness, feeling hopeless, and empty. You will have trouble finding pleasure and feel like your life is not worth living. This condition also affects your appetite and sleep, which puts you in an even worse situation. Your energy comes from the foods you consume, and when you're neglecting your diet, you are also depriving yourself of the source of your life energy. You become energetically depleted.

The crown chakra, when out of balance, produces a feeling of loneliness. In extreme situations, this can lead to suicidal thoughts, and eventually suicide. When you are feeling depressed, focus on working on balancing your heart chakra first. Your heart chakra helps you open up to love. It helps you open up to the sense of safety. It also helps you accept the idea that you are worthy of unconditional love and that there's nothing that you have to do to deserve it. Your crown chakra, which should only be treated when the root chakra is in good shape, is now in need of love. To work on your crown chakra, devote to religious, mindful, or spiritual practices. You should work on your relationship with the Divine, in whichever ways you practice spiritual beliefs.

Make sure to address any unconscious anger towards God. Most people find it hard to grasp that while God is a cosmic force that teaches you about right and wrong, He is also endlessly forgiving. When people feel guilty, they also feel like God thinks they are guilty, and God is judging them. This is never true. The Divine force is the force of unconditional forgiveness. If you feel angry with God, you actually feel angry at yourself. You assume that God is angry at you because you didn't act according to his/her/its teachings. In this case, you should con- template on God's imminent and unconditional love for every person. You can do this by reading scriptures or talking to a religious teacher who will explain how the Divine looks at people, and why it always forgives.

Grief

Loss can cause constriction and the closing of the heart chakra. Grief is a feeling that results from losing something that is precious to us. With relationships, jobs, and material goods, it's easier to cope with grief because there is a lesser significance to the loss. However, some losses, like the death of loved ones and children are very hard to cope with. There's no replacement for what we're missing, and relief seems impossible to find. Loss can very easily block your heart chakra, causing you to grief for a long time. This causes the feeling of loneliness, hopeless- ness, and the cultivation of bitterness. Grief is commonly followed by isolation. In some cases, isolation is a good idea for you to rejuvenate and pick yourself up. However, if isolation results from the unwillingness to reconnect with the world, it can become harmful.

Your heart chakra connects you to the sense of self-love and love for others. Grief can cause you to lose faith in love, and even choose to detach from it, to avoid feeling pain. The cure for grief is reconnecting with your own inner feeling of self-love, love for others, and the outside world. If you feel like grief has become toxic for you, there are many healthy ways for you to reconnect. You can start by practicing self-love and self-care and then move to connect with people, plants, and animals. If a heartbreak makes it hard for you to reconnect with your loved ones, you can start by connecting with plants and animals. Gradually, this connection will help you open up to connecting with people.

Guilt

An overwhelming feeling of guilt may constrict your solar plexus and the sacral plexus chakra. When you feel profoundly guilty of having done something wrong, whether or not this perception is true, you detach yourself from feeling pleasure. You deny yourself pleasure because you feel undeserving of it. This can cause you to repress your sexuality, emotions, and overall detach from doing things that make you happy. Guilt results in the loss of will to express yourself in healthy ways. To heal guilt, practice meditations for solar and sacral plexus chakras, and also work on healthy self-expression. Healing from guilt means being able to assume the responsibility for your actions but releasing the feeling of inadequacy. No one benefits from you feeling guilty. The guilt itself doesn't repair any harm that you may have done. You can work towards amending whatever harm you have done if there's room for it. If not, you can only work to learn from your mistakes. However, making a mistake doesn't mean that you no longer deserve to be happy.

Anxiety

Anxiety affects all chakras depending on the type of strain you're exposed to. Everyday life often entails a moderate amount of anxiety. However, long-term anxiety followed by constant stress can have a negative impact on your health. You will become more vulnerable to triggers. Within minutes of a triggering situation, you can find yourself in a state of panic. Most often, anxiety affects your crown and heart chakra. This happens when you start to feel like God doesn't have your back. The third eye chakra causes anxiety due to fear of the un- known, and distrust of your intuition.

This can severely impact your quality of life. When your throat chakra is out of harmony, you will be anxious about expressing your opinions and holding your truth. As a result, everything you have to say and the things that burdens you will be repressed. Holding on to past hurts can block your heart chakra and cause anxiousness because you feel disconnected from your own feelings. Intimidation and overwhelming fear, be it in the area of work, finance, or relationships, with the added pressure to perform perfectly, causes your solar plexus chakra to fall out of balance.

With sacral plexus chakra, anxiety results from feeling guilty and ashamed to confess your needs and insecurities. Over time, these built-up tensions can have a profoundly debilitating impact on your life. Anxiety also touches your root chakra in the form of feeling insecure and unsafe. To heal anxiety using chakra healing, you should examine your insecurities in all aspects of your inner being, starting from the bottom to the top. Screen all of your chakras and determine which areas are a source of negative energy. Then, start by practicing grounding to insure yourself that the Earth is supporting you. Proceed to heal your chakras using meditation, crystals, and essential oils. Focus on releasing your fears in regard to all issues that are relevant to the chakras.

Anger

Anger mostly affects your root chakra, but it also touches on the other energy centers as well. Anger, in its core, is a healthy feeling that drives you to stand up for yourself, establish boundaries, act, and initiate change. However, anger can also become a tool for you to repress sadness. When this happens, you are using anger to defend yourself from the inner feeling of sadness and hopelessness. Fear can also be the root of anger and your using anger away to the fence yourself being afraid. While anger resonates deeply with the root chakra, it affects all other chakras. If you are angry at God for the suffering of bad faith, this touches on your crown chakra.

Your third eye also becomes affected because due to this, you lose faith in your own intuition. You're out of touch with an inner sense of emotional intelligence. You will become unable to trust yourself, and as a result, you no longer trust the world and the Divine. You also start to distrust your community and your loved ones. The key to healing anger is to inspect the underlying feelings. For example, if you are angry for not standing up for yourself, the solution might be in balancing your solar plexus chakra. However, if you feel anger, to defend yourself from fear and sadness, the solutions are to treat your heart chakra and your sacral chakra. These chakras open you up to forgiveness and love.

If your anger roots in feeling burdened, then it's possible that you are holding in some truths that need to be said. These truths can relate to many areas of your life, from unpleasant things that you need to admit to yourself to deeply hidden truths you want to reveal to the world. If guilt and shame stop you from doing this, you need to learn how to overcome them. Only when you start going through life fully authentic to your inner truth will you be able to relieve the anger and live in peace.

Fear

Fear often links to anxiety. It results from the imbalance in the solar plexus and the root chakra. Being in constant fear means feeling like you are always in danger, and something will harm you if you don't pay close attention. You are constantly in fight-or-flight mode. While fear is a useful mechanism to protect yourself from danger, being constantly afraid is unhealthy. A state of chronic fear can start in situations when your basic needs are not being met. After a traumatic experience, you become unable to feel safe again. In the modern world, constant fear can arise from short episodes in your life when you lacked money, or there was a risk of poverty. You were probably taught to fear poverty and feel like you have to keep yourself safe to avoid starvation. This fear can become unconscious, always keeping you in a state of alert.

The imbalance of the solar plexus chakra results from the imbalances in the root chakra, which results from the lack of feeling supported in your basic needs. Unconscious fear can result from feeling unsupported in your childhood. For example, if your caregivers didn't shelter you from their personal struggles and they didn't create a sheltered environment, but instead have discussed their money problems in front of you, you may have grown up with a never-ending sense of endangerment.

As a child, your parents should have made you feel safe. Even if they struggled to put food on the table, you should have not been made aware of it. You were very young and unable to understand that these struggles are only temporary. To you, they were a lesson that life is scary, and the world is unsafe. Being a young child meant that you needed stable people around you to make you feel safe, fed, loved and sheltered.

If not, regardless of your current situation, you might still feel deeply unsafe. To recover from this, you can practice numerous rooting and grounding techniques. You can also focus on meditations that revolve around surrendering to the power of the Universe and enforcing the belief in inner security. Your ultimate goal is to feel unconditionally supported without the need for exterior manifestation. Grounding should be one of your main goals because the basic sense of security means feeling like the ground is physically supporting you. You can also contemplate more abstract ideas on how Divine forces always have your back and protect you from harm.

Stress

Stress affects your root chakra and all other chakras within your system. Stress results from demanding circumstances and putting your body and mind in a state of chronic strain that is physical, emotional, and mental. Cortisol, the main hormone of stress, is released during stress, as well as adrenaline. These hormones serve an initial purpose to help you get out of a threatening situation. However, being in this state for long periods of time causes you to gradually lose the ability to return to balance. Stress affects the crown chakra by isolating you from the Divine. It affects the throat chakra if you feel unable to express yourself. Stress also constricts the heart chakra, because it disconnects you from yourself and others. All of this may result in the feeling of low self-worth, which can close the solar plexus chakra.

The built-up feelings also burden your sacral plexus chakra and you stop expressing creativity. The initial steps to healing from stress include the grounding and healing of your root chakra. You need to return to caring for your own sense of security, safety, and the feeling that all of your basic needs will be met. This serves to relieve fear. Next, you want to work your way up through the chakras, addressing how stress and overwhelming circumstances have affected your system, other chakras, and other aspects of your personality.

Back pain

Pains in the area of your upper, middle, and lower back that haven't resulted from any physical trauma or physical stress may result from imbalances in your chakra system. Upper-back pains are often rooted in the imbalance of the throat and heart Chakra. They are physical manifestations of closing yourself off to love and truth. If you are isolated from feeling love and you have difficulty ex- pressing it, it can manifest physically in the form of back pain. Middle-back pains relate to your heart chakra and the solar plexus chakra. When you have issues receiving love, accepting that you deserve love, and living according to that truth, you can start harboring secret pain and rage. As you hide these feelings from yourself, they have no other way to surface but through the pain. Pain in your lower back may result from the imbalance in your route and sacral plexus chakra.

Whenever you feel confined, like something isn't available to you, whether it's abundance, love, or relationships; the energy inside your root chakra and the sacral plexus chakra constricts. Technically, this type of pain results from limiting yourself in expressing desires. If there is no physical cause to your lower back pain, it may have resulted from unconsciously forbidding yourself to express physical and emotional needs. This can happen due to guilt and shame. Denying yourself the right to express needs and desires can be related both to emotional and sexual needs. Often, these two dimensions intertwine. The root of this limitation can be in feeling undeserving of pleasantness due to something that you have done in the past. To overcome this and heal the lower back pain, screen yourself for shame and guilt in various areas of your life. The purpose of this is to admit your feelings to yourself, process them instead of suppressing them.

Hip pain

Pain in your hips can result from suppressed feelings related to avoidance. This pain resonates with the sacral plexus chakra. Whenever you suppress feelings in a stressful situation, tension can build up in your sacral plexus chakra. Your sacral plexus chakra is the place where you admit your own feelings to yourself and empower yourself to become vulnerable and express them. If you've limited yourself against expressing feelings of vulnerability, like the need for intimacy, anger, hurt, or the issues with abandonment and intimacy, all of this tension could have built up in your sacral plexus chakra. To relieve the pain in your lower back, work around opening yourself to vulnerability, and acknowledge that you have the right to reach out for support. You also need to learn how to treat yourself with more com- passion and stop shaming yourself. Whenever you feel weak and vulnerable, meditations that revolve around self-compassion and acceptance are helpful to balance your sacral plexus chakra.

Jaw pain

Pain in your jaw can result from the imbalance in the throat chakra. As you know by now, your throat chakra is the place of hearing, admitting, and speaking your truth. If you haven't been doing this, you might have created an energetic and emotional blockage in the area of your throat. The pain might be occurring be-because you are refusing to hear your truth. The only way for your mind and body to signal this to you is through the pain.

So, how do you heal jaw pain? You bring everything that you have been avoiding to say to awareness. Practice speaking the truth and look into the truth that you may be avoiding to admit to yourself.

Leg pain

Leg pain often results from the energy blockage in the sacral solar plexus, and the root chakra. As you know by now, your root chakra is in charge of feeling safe, while your solar plexus chakra is in charge of feeling strong. When you don't feel safe and you don't feel strong, that means you feel frightened and weak. It means you feel powerless. If you have unexplainable leg pain, it means that you may have been avoiding to confront feeling powerless. The feeling of powerlessness is often associated with thoughts of not having enough control. However, no one is truly in control of anything. Your path to healing from psychosomatic leg pain is working to ground yourself and tap into your own spiritual power, instead of looking for the outside manifestations of it.

Shift your mind from trying to manifest your power externally, and work to feel it spiritually. Aside from grounding and balancing your chakras with meditation, crystals, and essential oils, track your behaviors and actions to see how your unconscious patterns of behavior serve to establish control in your life. Your legs may simply be over- tired because you're always running around in the efforts to avoid losing control. You may feel like your life will fall apart if you're not always on top of everything.

Healing with Chakra Chants & Sounds

Sounds can heal and balance your chakras, too. Just like colors, sounds have distinct wavelengths and frequencies to which the seven energy centers respond to. The therapeutic sounds include the ones you create and the sounds from your surroundings. Think of songs, chants, prayers, music and the sounds present in natural landscapes such as oceans, forests and meadows. Sound healing or therapy has been employed in Western, Oriental and African cultures since the ancient times.

These days, healing sounds and music are used primarily for relaxation, whether you have a medical condition or are simply under stress. However, the belief that sounds have chakra healing and balancing properties comes from early Chinese, Tibetan and Indian medicines. There are different ways to heal and balance your chakras with the help of sounds. The most notable ones are: chakra toning and bija mantras. There are also various tools whose sounds can benefit the energy centers in your body.

Chakra Toning

Chakra toning is a technique that makes use of vowel sounds to clear and balance the energy centers. You can do this every day to be more familiar with the natural harmonics from the vowels. In speech, there is a thing called information energy. The vowels work as the carriers of information energy while the consonants are the breakers of the energy flow. In ancient Chinese, Hebrew and Sanskrit, vowels are also deemed as sacred because they bear the focus and intention in speech. Before you begin toning your chakras, you should find a place where no one can disturb you and where you cannot disturb anyone. You should also get rid of possible sources of noises such as gadgets, clocks and running appliances.

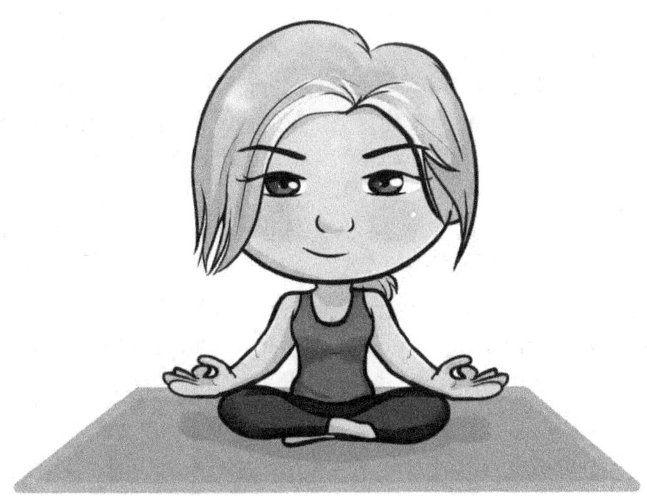

Step 1: To start, sit comfortably on the floor or ground. You may use a mat or cushion. Keep your back straight to facilitate uninterrupted energy flow from one chakra to another. It also helps to visualize your head floating above a cord and your body hanging below.

Step 2: Before you make the sounds, channel your focus, energy and intent to each chakra. Take a deep breath. Let your lower stomach expand as you inhale.

Step 3: Gently utter the sounds. It is up to you to decide the frequency. When you make the sounds, feel your body for resonance except for the throat because it will always vibrate to get the right pitch. The right pitch differs every now and then. It actually depends on a variety of factors such as diet, mood, personality and personal activities. Do it slowly and calmly. Do not strain your voice.

- For the root chakra, utter your deepest "UUH" sound akin to the vowel sound of "cup".
- For the sacral chakra, utter an "OOO" sound that is similar to the vowel sound of the word "you". In terms of pitch, this is slightly higher than the guttural sound for the first chakra.
- For the solar plexus chakra, utter an "OH" sound that is like the vowel sound for the word "go". This is also a higher pitched version of the previous tone.
- For the heart chakra, utter an "AH" sound. The said sound deemed as an embodiment of passion which is an aspect of the heart chakra.

- For the throat chakra, utter an "EYE" sound that is similar to the vowel sound in "me". Do not make the mistake of associating the said sound to your third eye chakra.
- For the third eye chakra, utter an "AYE" sound that is like the vowel sound in "say".
- For the crown chakra, utter the highest "EEE" sound you can produce. Interestingly, when you try to tone from the "UUH" to "EEH" sounds quickly and continuously, you will notice that it forms the word "why".

Step 4: Visualize the energy in each breath to come into your body and pass through your target chakra.

Step 5: Once you are done, sit still for at least 10 minutes for the energy to sink in to your chakras. When you feel dizzy afterwards, probably due to the prolonged sitting, tone an extensive "aaaah" sound to direct the energy back to your heart chakra. Then tone using an extensive "ooooh" sound to drive it to your lower chakras.

CONCLUSION

Learning about chakras is a journey that everyone should take at some point in life. The lessons you learn are useful and will help you change the course of your life. Mastery of your chakras is important in that it accords you an infinite understanding of your spirituality and its connection to the universe around you. What is interesting about chakras is that they are things we know about, but never pay attention to. Most of the time you go about your life like a blind person, unaware of the energy around you, or the energy you emit. Ever wondered why you keep attracting bad company while other people attract good company?

In Sanskrit, you attract similar energy to the one you emit. If you constantly give off negative vibes, you will attract negativity. Those who give off positive energies always have positivity around them. You want nothing but good things in your life. It is time for you to embrace your spirituality, learn about your chakras, and how they affect or control your life. From the first to the last chakra, so much happens in your life that you should learn about.

The exercises and routines recommended for balancing your chakras are easy to perform. Allow yourself a few minutes each day for this, and you can get your life back in line. To live and enjoy your life with all the happiness that the universe bestows upon you, the secret lies in a mastery of the seven chakras. Mastery means you understand what they do, and how they control your life. This level of mastery will help you improve your relationships with people around you, your relationships with nature and the entire universe. Balanced chakras give you peace, not just with people around you, but more importantly, peace with yourself. After all, you cannot know how to love and care for others until you to learn how to do the same for yourself, and the value it holds in your life.

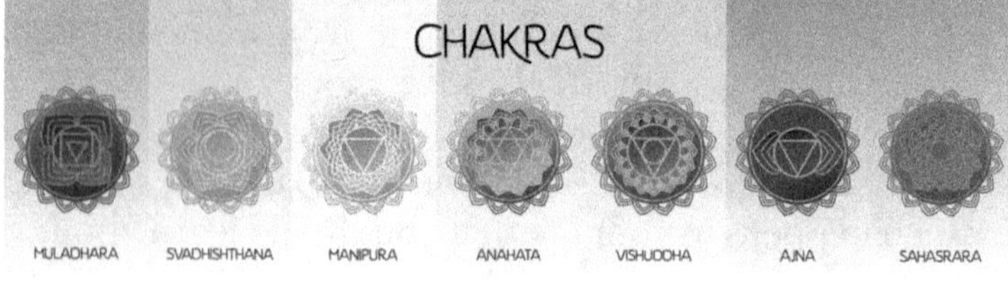